Introducing
The Masterson Method™

BEYOND
HORSE MASSAGE

A Breakthrough Interactive Method for Alleviating Soreness, Strain and Tension

By USET Endurance Team Equine Massage Therapist
JIM MASTERSON with Stefanie Reinhold

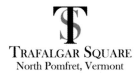

TRAFALGAR SQUARE
North Pomfret, Vermont

First published in 2011 by
Trafalgar Square Books
North Pomfret, Vermont 05053

Printed in China

Library of Congress Cataloging-in-Publication Data
Masterson, Jim.
   Beyond horse massage : a breakthrough interactive method for alleviating soreness, stress, and tension /
Jim Masterson with Stefanie Reinhold ; foreword by McLain Ward
      p. cm.
   Includes bibliographical references and index.
   ISBN 978-1-57076-472-1 (hardcover)
1. Horses—Diseases—Alternative treatment—Handbooks, manuals, etc. 2. Massage for animals—Handbooks, manuals, etc. 3. Veterinary physical therapy—Handbooks, manuals, etc. 4. Horses—Health—Handbooks, manuals, etc. 5. Horses—Effect of stress on—Handbooks, manuals, etc. 6. Stress (Physiology)—Handbooks, manuals, etc. 7. Stress management—Handbooks, manuals, etc. I. Reinhold, Stefanie. II. Title.
   SF951.M425 2011
   636.1'089--dc23
                         2011030823

The photograph on p. 159 is by Lori McIntosh Photography.

All other photographs by Marcus Brauer (www.pferdehessen.de) *except:* pp. 14, 15, 28, 29, 59, 76, 87 *bottom,* 89, 90 *left,* 115, 122, 128 *right,* 157 (Geof Northridge); pp. 8, 9, 10, 40, 41 *top,* 47 *bottom,* 56, 82 *bottom,* 86, 99, 131, 149 *top,* 150, 156 (Joseph Stanski); pp 5, 24, 33, 62, 104, 143 (Stefanie Reinhold); p. 145 (from *Tug of War: Classical versus Modern Dressage* by Dr. Gerd Heuschmann and used by permission of the publisher); pp. 4, 49 (Tamara Yates); p. 139 (Leona Reinhold).

Illustrations from: *The Horse's Muscles in Motion* by Sarah Wyche and used by permission of the publisher (pp. 64 *top,* 105 *bottom,* 106, 107, 108, 109, 110, 152); *Tug of War: Classical versus Modern Dressage* by Dr. Gerd Heuschmann and used by permission of the publisher (pp. 35, 64 *bottom*).

Book design by Lauryl Eddlemon
Cover design by RM Didier
Typeface: Myriad

10 9 8 7 6

This, my first book, is dedicated to

my parents, who by their approach to life taught me
how to live outside the box,

my partner and wife Conley, who keeps me going,

and of course to,
The Horse, whatever else can be said about it.

Contents

Foreword

I first met Jim Masterson at the 2006 World Equestrian Games in Aachen, Germany. Sometimes it can be stressful to have new people working on your horse the last two weeks before a big event, but Jim has such a relaxed demeanor around horses (and riders) that all the US Endurance Team members were actually vying for his time. The horses clearly love Jim's techniques, and the result is better range of motion with a reduced risk of injury. (An added benefit is that watching him work on a horse actually relaxes the observer, too!)

Unfortunately Jim and I live in different parts of the country so I do not get to see him nearly enough, but I have had the great fortune to work with him at all the world championships since that first time in Germany—and at several other major rides in between. Jim is always a huge asset, both because of his skills in massage and his willingness to jump in and help in any way he can. He is the epitome of "team player," and—as you'll find in his book—his sense of humor is fabulous!

Beyond Horse Massage offers the reader a window into Jim's work and allows clear access to his unique body of knowledge. With this book, Jim has given us the tools to support our horses in ways most of us could previously only imagine. He has empowered us to maximize performance by improving flexibility. The end result is reduced susceptibility to injuries, as well as heightened performance. But his methods can be used for other purposes, as well. His bodywork is a powerful tool for speeding recovery after strenuous workouts, and its use significantly reinforces the rider's/trainer's relationship with the horse.

Meg Sleeper, VMD, DACVIM (Cardiology)
Member United States Endurance Squad
2004, 2006, 2008, 2010

Preface

When I first began working with competition horses I was hauling and grooming horses for a show barn on the A-level hunter-jumper circuit in the Midwest. Before this, I had never had an interest in massage or physical therapy of any kind—human or animal.

This all changed while at a spring horse show in Estes Park, Colorado. Our trainer hired two equine massage therapists to work on our horses. They started their massage by going very gently with their hands over an area of the horse called the *bladder meridian*. This exercise was to relax the horse before the actual muscle work began. I was fascinated by the subtle responses in the horse's eyes, lips, and breathing as they slowly ran their hands lightly over him. Although the horse was certainly relaxed by the time they were done, I noticed that there was a definite correlation between where their hands were on the horse, the changes in the horse's eyes (for example), and other subtle responses of the horse during this process.

I suggested to the trainer that she hire these two wonderful and very sensitive massage therapists to spend a few hours teaching me some basics of equine massage that I could use on our barn's horses, at the shows and at home. Having virtually no other training in massage, to guide my work I relied mainly on paying attention to what the horse was telling me through his subtle

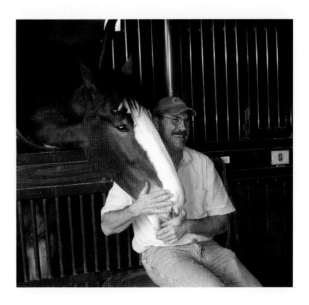

responses. Fascinated by the reaction to very light input, I applied very subtle levels of touch, waiting to see what would happen. I found that I could get a response from the horse with almost no contact at all. By being patient (lazy), watching what was going on with the horse, and adjusting the levels of pressure (or no pressure), I found that the horse would give larger and larger visual responses that correlated with softening and releases of tension in the areas I was working on.

As my goal was to improve movement and mobility more than to work with the muscle itself, I began to apply movement to this method of releasing tension in the horse. I found that by staying under the horse's threshold of bracing and resistance, I could find restriction and then ask for movement in a way that allowed the horse to release the tension in an area. He would then let me know he had released the tension with large release responses, such as repeated yawning, snorting, and sneezing, and rolling back the second eyelid. This interaction with the horse turned out to be not only fun, but effective.

I also had the benefit of working in the highly competitive environment of show jumping. I was fortunate to have access to valuable feedback from talented trainers, riders, veterinarians, and equine therapists—not to mention the horses. With this feedback, I was able to determine what specific areas of the horse consistently accumulated tension in work, which when released, showed improvement in performance.

As I gained more clients, the interactive, intuitive, and results-oriented nature of this bodywork began to attract the attention of horse owners interested not only in performance but in relationship, communication, and the bond of trust that develops with the horse. The results could actually be seen as the work was being done on the horse. I began showing interested owners what to look for, and how to apply basic techniques. This soon led to the making of an instructional DVD, *Equine Massage for Performance Horses: The Masterson Method™*, then to demonstrations for riding clubs and barns. In 2005 I began teaching Weekend Seminar Workshops around the country and began getting requests from people in Europe and Australia who had bought the DVD from our website: www.mastersonmethod.com.

We now teach seminars and courses around the United States and Europe. This interest in learning how to read what is going on with the horse coincides with the precepts of natural horsemanship and resistance-free training so popular today. The interest of horse people who want both performance and improved relationship with their horses has led to the development of two learning paths in the Masterson Method: one for horse lovers and horse owners, and a professional learning path for equine-massage and bodywork therapists interested in learning or integrating the Masterson Method into their practice. This book is an introduction to both. Once the basic principles of using the horse's responses to touch are felt and learned, then the techniques taught in this book can be applied to the entire horse, applied individually to specific issues, or used simply to connect and build trust with your horse.

The Masterson Method is something you do *with* the horse, rather than *to* the horse. Whether you are someone whose appreciation for horses motivates you to learn as much as you can about these wonderful creatures, a serious competitor in equine sports, or a dedicated professional in equine care and well-being, this is something that you can easily learn to directly benefit you and your horse.

PART ONE

The Masterson Method™

INTEGRATED EQUINE
PERFORMANCE BODYWORK

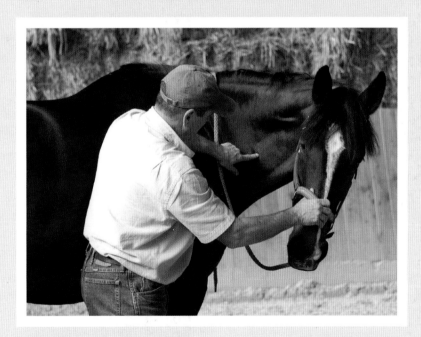

1

CHAPTER 1

What Is the Masterson Method?

The Masterson Method—Integrated Equine Performance Bodywork—is a unique, interactive method of equine bodywork in which you learn to recognize and use the responses of the horse to your touch to find and release accumulated tension in key junctions of the body that most affect performance. In contrast to most traditional modalities, it enables the horse to *actively participate* in the process of releasing tension. It is something you do *with* the horse, rather than *to* the horse. This participation and interaction is what makes the method fascinating for those who use it. In fact, *if you do not allow the horse to participate, it does not work!*

Although this bodywork was developed to improve performance in equine athletes competing in high-demand environments such as show jumping, harness racing, endurance, reining, and barrel racing, its intuitive and interactive nature can help to not only improve performance, but to access a new level of communication with the horse.

The results of this interaction are both visual and palpable *(you can feel with your hand):*

- Visual signs of release of tension in the horse's body.
- Improved performance, suppleness, mobility, and comfort.
- And most importantly, the immediate bond of trust that begins to develop as a result of this cooperation.

This is a very practical, hands-on approach that you can begin using immediately. You do not have to have knowledge of anatomy or massage to begin using the basic techniques of this method. The techniques you will need are easily learned with the help of this book. The principles of touch and response will be demonstrated to you by the horse from the very beginning. Once the basic techniques are learned, and you follow what the horse is telling you, the horse lets you know where tension is stored, guides you in releasing that tension, and lets you know when it is released. The results are real time.

This approach can be easily integrated into other modalities, so it can be of value to the professional massage and bodywork therapist as well. Once learned, these tools enhance effectiveness of other modalities through immediate feedback from the horse. Another tool for the professional toolbox!

The Techniques used in this method can be used together, from front to hind on the horse, or individual Techniques can be used to address particular issues on different areas of the horse's body. As the results are visible and immediate, many of these Techniques will yield visible and immediate improvements to specific performance-related issues.

That said, you will soon see while working with this method how interconnected different areas of the horse are, and not just because I say so (not a very convincing reason) but because the horse will show you. When working on one area of the horse you will often get a "visible" release in another area. How these areas are interconnected and how they affect performance makes logical sense once you look at the anatomy. Anatomical explanations will accompany the Techniques presented in this book, and a quick reference chart relating specific Techniques to common performance issues will follow in the Appendix.

HOW DOES IT WORK?

Survival Instinct and the Horse's Language

One reason this method works so well is because of the horse's incredible awareness and sensitivity to outside stimuli. This is how he survives. Working *with* this sensitivity you can access a level of the horse's nervous system that enables him to release deep stress in his muscles, connective tissue and structure. To do this you must learn how to use touch, and how to read what the horse is telling you through his responses and body language.

To fully understand this, you need to be aware of a couple of underlying principles of the horse's survival instincts:

a) Prey Animal
As a *prey animal,* the horse's survival in nature depends on his ability to flee from danger.

Getting away from danger, intrusion or discomfort is the horse's *first survival response.* If he doesn't have this option, as is normally the case when with humans, the horse's *second survival response* is to "brace," "push," or "guard against" intrusion, discomfort, or pain. This is the survival response that you learn to bypass.

By applying Techniques at levels of pressure that *don't* trigger this bracing survival response, (whether it's internal or external), and knowing from the horse's responses when this is happening, you can bypass the bracing response and access that part of the nervous system that will release tension.

By nature, most horses take the path of least resistance when given the option—and when asked properly—and this path is for him to release tension.

b) Herd Animal
As a *herd* animal the horse relies, to a large part, on body language for communication in the herd. This can be seen from the most obvious flattening of ears and baring of teeth, to the slightest softening of the eye, shift of weight, change in breathing, and even subtler signs.

The horse will instinctively do its best not to show outward signs of pain or weakness, to prevent himself from being either picked out of the herd by a predator or kicked out of the herd as a weak link. This is why it is so often challenging to accurately evaluate lameness in the horse.

When you learn to follow the signs and responses the horse gives you, he lets you know when you are being effective, where he is holding tension, and when his body has released this hidden tension. By using levels of pressure that the horse's defense system doesn't internally resist—knowing how to read and work with the horse when this is happening—you enable the horse's nervous system to release tension that he has been covering up.

A fascinating aspect of this is that when the horse begins to realize that you are allowing him to release tension that he has been holding instinctively, he begins to take part in the process by more readily showing you release responses, and letting go of tension in his body more easily. *This creates a deeper bond of trust between you and your horse* (fig.1.1).

The Junctions of the Body That Most Affect Performance

Repetitive work, pain, lameness, or compensation for any discomfort can cause tension patterns to develop in muscles and connective tissue that can restrict movement in joints and major junctions of the body. This accumulated tension and restricted movement can negatively affect performance, comfort, add to psychological and emotional strain, and result in a loss of willingness and behavior problems. These restrictive tension patterns can themselves eventually contribute to lameness. Even after the primary cause of lameness is removed, the tension patterns and restriction often remain. A point has been reached where the horse cannot completely release this tension without help. The purpose of this method is to help the horse release accumulated stress and tension in the body that he cannot release on his own.

In the Masterson Method, you begin by focusing on the *three main junctions* of the body that most affect performance. These are:

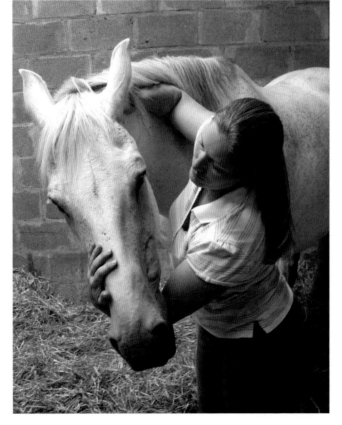

1.1 The deeper bond of trust between human and horse.

- **The Poll-Atlas Junction**
- **The Neck-Shoulder-Withers (Cervical-Thoracic C7-T1) Junction**
- **The Hind-End (Sacroiliac) Junction**

When tension is released in any of these key junctions, tension is released in muscles and connective tissue in the larger areas of that junction, and often in more remote areas of the horse's body.

The most important junction in relation to overall mobility and comfort in the horse is the *Poll-Atlas Junction.* In my experience, tension, pain, or discomfort anywhere in the horse's body shows up as tension in the poll.

The other two main junctions are where the horse's limbs join the body. Here, forces exerted by the horse's limbs as well as concussion during movement are transferred to the body. Tension accumulates in these junctions as a result. When tension patterns begin to accumulate unilaterally, meaning more to one side than the other, forces

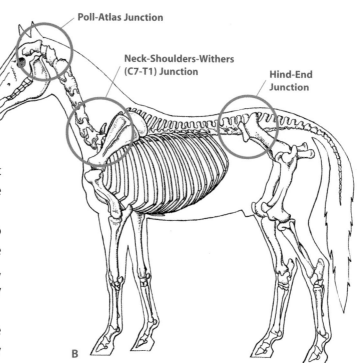

are exerted in an unbalanced manner and performance problems can become apparent in bending, lead changes, and movement. This potential imbalance applies to all three main junctions. It's important to remember that you release tension in these junctions because it has been shown by the horse that it works.

Touch and Response— An Intuitive Approach

"Touch" and "Response," when you get right down to it, are nothing more than *stimulus* and *behavior.*

When you apply the correct stimulus (touch), you will get the correct behavior (response), which starts the process of *release* in the horse. When you use the correct level of *touch* and can

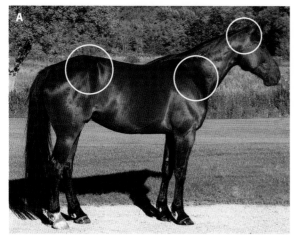

1.2 A & B **The three main junctions of the horse.**

recognize the responses that correlate to what you are doing, you can follow those responses to a successful release of tension by the horse.

Although this sounds scientific so far, once you start to recognize the responses of the horse and you get the correlation between what you are doing and what the horse is saying, the horse begins to guide the process.

The more you pay attention to what the horse is saying, the more you begin to recognize subtler responses from the horse to the point that you begin to "feel" as much as see what is going on. You often start to sense that an area is about to release before the horse visibly shows you the release. It soon becomes less about *seeing* and *thinking,* and more about *feeling.* The horse begins to participate by responding more readily and learns to release tension more easily.

Defined Levels of Touch— Less Is More

One of the distinctions between the Masterson Method and traditional massage is the role the horse plays in the process. With traditional massage you are trained with your hands to find— then "go to work" on—tension and anomalies in the muscle, using levels of pressure that will break them up.

With this method, you listen to what the horse's body has to say and adjust your pressure to get the result you want: the *release* from the horse. If there is any question about whether you are using the correct amount of pressure, the answer almost always is "less is more." The levels of pressure you use can range from almost noth-ing to about as much pressure as you can apply, depending on which area you are working on and what the horse is telling you.

To avoid the use of technical terms (pounds/square inch, for example) in describing what level to use in any particular exercise, and to make it easy to visualize, we have developed the more palpable descriptions below (that suspiciously, as someone pointed out in a seminar, have mostly to do with food). The key is to let the horse's initial response, or lack of response, let you know if you are using too much pressure.

The following five terms are used to describe the different levels of pressure you apply during the bodywork exercises:

- *Air Gap*—Barely touching the surface. If you were to run your hand lightly down your arm, you would be barely brushing across the hairs on your arm.

- *Egg Yolk*—This is the amount of pressure it would take to barely indent a raw egg yolk with your fingertip. It might be a good idea to break an egg in a bowl to see how light this actually is.

- *Grape*—The amount of pressure it would take to indent a grape.

- *Soft Lemon*—The amount of pressure it would take to squeeze a soft, ripe lemon.

- *Hard Lime*—The amount of pressure it would take to squeeze a hard, unripe lime. In some cases this can be just about as hard as you can push.

It's easy to misjudge or miscalculate how much pressure you are using with these Techniques. This can happen when you are first applying the Techniques and your focus is on your body position and where to place your hands. However, *the level of touch you use is the single most important thing that will determine the level of success you will have!*

Don't despair! In each of the illustrated step-by-step sections you will find corresponding, detailed notes around the level of "feel" and "touch" needed to get the most out of the Technique. These will help you become most effective.

Practice your levels of touch on a friend who can give you feedback. During the course of our seminars, most students need to be reminded several times to lighten their touch. Since I will not be there to remind you as you learn and practice these Techniques, your mantra should always be, "Less is more."

This doesn't mean that you will not use any pressure or strength with these Techniques. It only means that you will need to keep in mind that, contrary to our human way of doing things, when you run into resistance to whatever level of pressure or touch you are using, when you soften or yield to that resistance, it will allow the horse to release that tension (fig. 1.3).

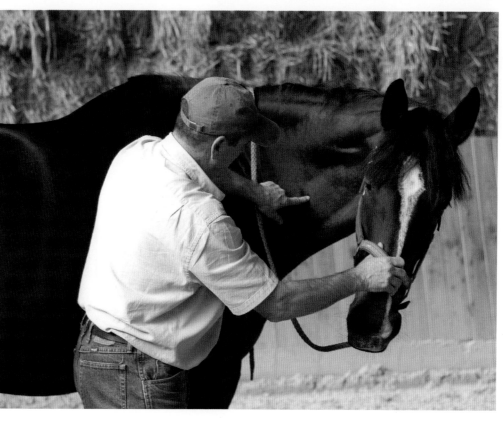

1.3 Use different levels of pressure.

Types of Responses

The correct level of touch will put your horse in a relaxed frame of mind enabling him to more easily tell you through his responses when you have successfully helped him release tension. Monitoring these responses continually will allow you to see where tension is stored, and see or feel when the horse lets go of tension. Even the degree of release can be read by the intensity of the horse's responses, in real time. As you practice these Techniques, you will find that very soon your recognition and use of these responses will become automatic and second nature.

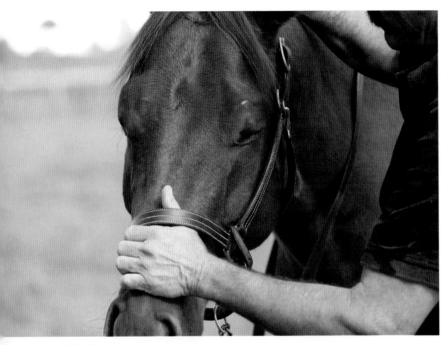

1.4 A Blinking.

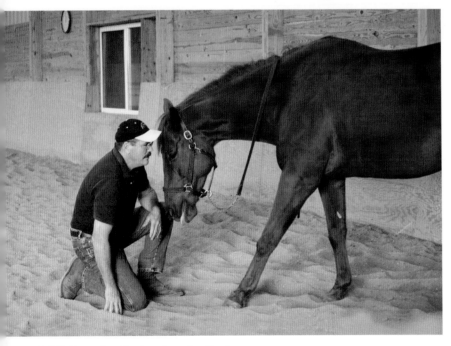

1.4 B Dropping the head, and softening.

Below are the visual responses you are looking for. They range from the subtlest responses to responses that are more obvious:

Subtle Responses

These are usually responses that demonstrate you are on an area of tension that the horse is blocking, and you are successfully using a level of pressure that is bypassing the horse's bracing survival response.

- Blinking or twitching of the eye (fig. 1.4 A)
- Twitching or quivering of the lips
- Change in breathing—holding breath, breathing faster
- Sighing, or letting out breath
- Dropping the head (fig.1.4 B)
- Softening of the eye, or facial expression (see fig.1.1, p. 4)

Larger Responses

These are usually responses that indicate some level of a release of tension in the horse.

They range from mild releases *(licking and chewing),* to large releases of accumulated tension and stress *(repeated yawning and rolling back the second eyelid).*

- Licking and chewing
- Snorting or sneezing—especially repeatedly—and sometimes grunting (fig.1.4 C)
- Shaking the head and body, "shaking loose"
- Yawning—especially repeatedly (fig. 1.4 D)
- Rolling back the second eyelid
- Stretching and flexing
- Fidgeting

Interesting notes and correlations on different responses:

Licking and chewing: Many horse trainers use licking and chewing as an indication of submission in a social or herd context. It has a similar significance in the neurological context—letting-go, yielding or releasing.

Snorting or sneezing: In warming up for work, many dressage riders know that the horse has loosened up in the back, or has warmed up enough to begin working when he drops his head and sneezes or snorts.

Shaking the head and shoulders, and stretching and flexing: Often, while I'm working on a horse, I will step back at regular intervals or when I feel the horse has released some tension to see what he has to say. Often, he will take a couple of seconds to feel what is going on in his body, then "shake loose" as I like to call it (fig. 1.5), or he'll reach around and scratch his foreleg or flank with his nose. I will step up and do some more work, then step back to see what he has to say, and he'll reach around a little farther to scratch his hip or rump. I'll do a little more work then step back and the horse will reach around even farther, and with his hind hoof scratch behind the ear. This happens too often to be just a coincidence. It's apparent that as the horse feels a release of restriction, he will reach around and stretch or flex the area that has released.

Repeated yawning and rolling back the second eyelid: This is the biggest indicator of a large

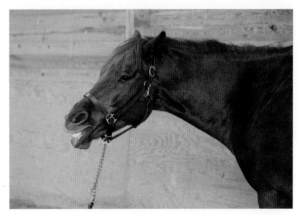
1.4 C Sneezing and snorting.

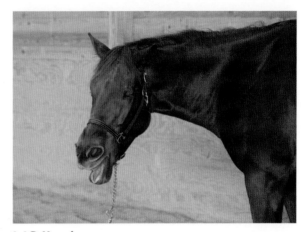
1.4 D Yawning.

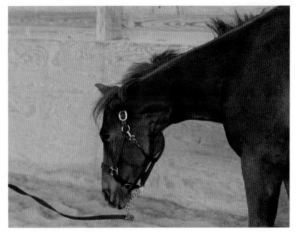
1.5 Shaking it out.

release of tension (fig. 1.6). You have to see it to experience the thrill of this release. And you will!

The importance of fidgeting: When I began working on horses this took a while for me to realize, and when I started teaching my method, one of

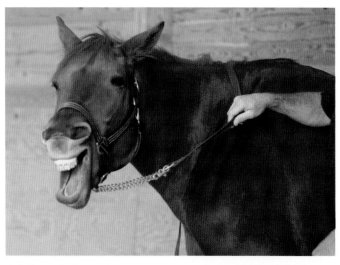

1.6 Repeated yawning.

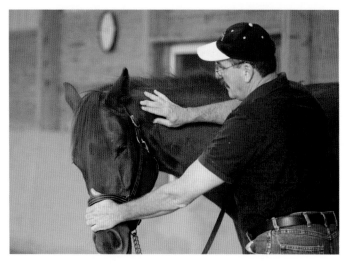

1.7 Look for the correlation between what you are doing and the behavior the horse is giving you in response.

the first questions that came from my students was, "What do I do when I am doing a particular Technique on a horse and he begins to fidget or move around?"

If you are using the method properly—meaning the horse is *relaxed* and not *bracing*—when he starts to fidget, walk or move, it is an indication that he is about to *release.*

What you do when this happens is stay softly with what you are doing for just a little longer. This means that you may have to move with the horse. Almost always, the horse will then show you a release response.

Connecting Touch to Response

So, you might say, "Horses *always* blink, yawn, lick their lips, fidget, and sometimes stretch. How do you tell if it is a response or if they are just chewing food, blinking at flies, scratching an itch, for example?"

The answer is that you are not just looking for these behaviors: *You are looking for the correlation between what you are doing with the horse in that moment, and the behavior the horse is giving you in response.* This is the key (fig. 1.7). All it takes is the patience to watch, wait, and see what the horse has to say about it, and the patience and willingness to go slowly and lightly with your touch. Remember, *less is more!*

Once you've learned to use the correct level of touch, to recognize the horse's responses, and to recognize the *correlation* between your touch and the horse's response, then following the steps I outline on the next few pages will get you started on this interactive journey.

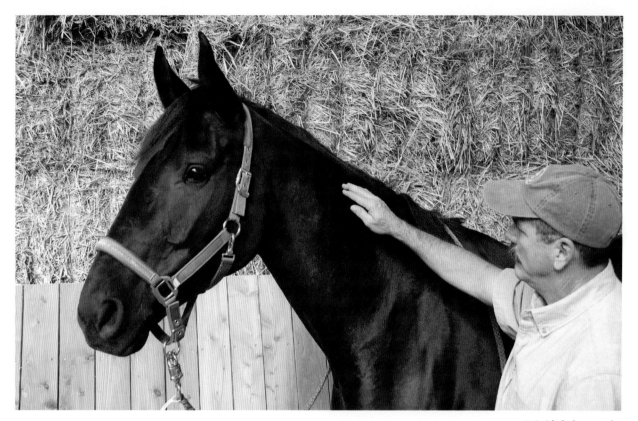

1.8 Lightly search.

Search, Response, Stay, Release

a) Search

Softly search with a light touch, closely watching the horse's responses (fig. 1.8).

b) Response

The horse responds to your touch (in this photo, by blinking) as you go over a spot or area of tension (fig.1.9).

c) Stay

Stay on that spot or area—continuing to watch the horse's responses—at a level of pressure that doesn't trigger an *internal bracing response*. This

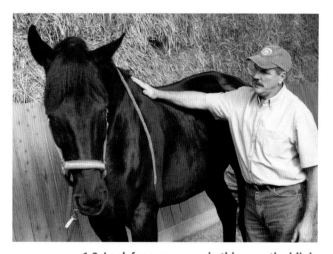

1.9 Look for a response, in this case, the blink.

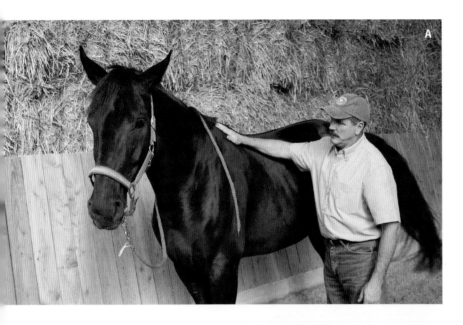

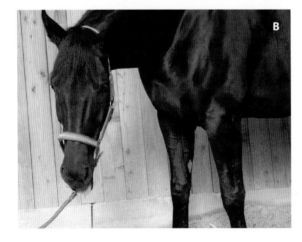

1.10 A & B Stay lightly on the spot (A), until you get a release, in this case a head drop and licking and chewing (B).

may take as little as a second, or as long as several minutes (figs. 1.10 A).

d) Release

Your horse shows a release response that signals release of tension in the area (fig. 1.10 B).

You use this *Search, Response, Stay, Release* process to:

- Find areas of hidden stress or tension *(Search, Response)*.
- Apply the correct level of touch to enable the horse to release *(Stay)*.
- Read the horse's response when a release has occurred *(Release)*.

By applying this process, the horse tells you:

- *Where* stress is accumulated.
- *How much* pressure is needed to release it.
- *When* it has been released.

This *Search, Response, Stay, Release* process applies when you are practicing Techniques using the lightest levels of touch and looking for the subtlest responses, to actually applying movement to the three main junctions (see p. 5) and getting visual and palpable responses.

Don't worry if this concept doesn't "feel right" quite yet. You will get it as you move through the hands-on chapters (beginning on p. 23).

The Importance of Going Slowly

In order for the horse to participate in this process, you must allow him to do so on *his* own time. Let go of the element of time or the horse won't respond. Throw away the clock. You are on the horse's agenda. Go slowly in the *Search,* watch for *Response,* and when you get one, *Stay, Stay, Stay* until you get a *Release,* or until you are sure there is nothing there.

Note: Different horses have different personalities. Some respond more readily than others. Some are more guarded and give you hardly anything, then after you have walked away, they will show the release. But there is almost always some kind of response, and soon you will get good at recognizing even the subtlest change that signifies progress.

Yielding and Using Sense of "Feel"

Initially, use a very light touch along an area of the horse called the *bladder meridian* (see chapter 4, p. 24). In addition to giving you information about where the horse is holding tension, this establishes the sensitivity of the horse and the level of touch you will use to start. It sets the stage for exercises that involve movement of different parts of the horse's body.

With these Techniques you will also be asking the horse to move his head, neck, legs, and body in ways and positions that will facilitate relaxation and release of tension.

You also use *Touch* and *Response* when asking for movement. In this case the *responses* can be *palpable* as well as *visual.* Using your hands to ask for movement is *Touch.* When you feel any resistance, the horse softening or yielding is *his Response.*

The Principle of Non-Resistance

How you ask the horse to move is fundamental to the success of this method. If the horse is not in a relaxed state when you ask for movement then he is, in a sense, *bracing* as he moves. *"Ask"* is the key word here. When you ask the horse to bend his

nose toward you, for example, and the horse resists, your first impulse is to pull harder *to make him* bend toward you. If you react to the resistance by countering it, the horse will continue to resist, tense, or brace. Even if he is still bringing his head toward you, the horse is still, to some degree, resisting, tensing, or bracing as he's moving.

Apply *the principle of non-resistance:* When the horse resists, soften your hand slightly so when he feels *you* stop pulling, he will let go, and *you* then continue the movement. When you give the horse *nothing* to resist, he will stop resisting, and you can immediately continue on with your move.

Here's another example: When you pick up the horse's foot and he pulls away, your first intuitive reaction may be to pull back. If you keep pulling it causes him to continue to pull away. However, if you yield or go with him just slightly, he will yield and relax. This doesn't mean you let go, only *soften*—or yield—to the resistance. Then, immediately ask him to continue with the movement. This may not make sense right now, but you'll be trying it out on a horse soon.

Exercises to Understand the Principle of Non-Resistance

■ **Ask the horse to move forward and back.**
When you use a lead rope to ask the horse to move forward you can use mechanical force to pull him forward or you can use the *principle of non-resistance.*

To do this, apply very gentle pressure (the slightest pressure possible) to the lead rope and as the horse yields the slightest bit by moving his nose forward slightly or even shifting his weight—release pressure and ask immediately

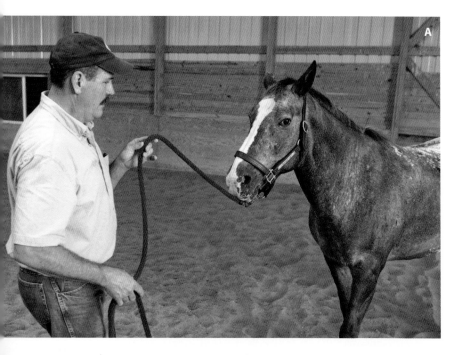

again for another yield (figs. 1.11 A & B). Ask, release, ask, release. You can ask a little more each time until he shifts his weight completely and takes a step.

■ **Ask him to move his hind end to the side.**
Use the same Technique to ask the horse to move his hind end. Apply slight pressure with your fingers to the rump or hip (fig. 1.12 A). When there is the slightest yield, soften your pressure, then ask again (fig. 1.12 B). Resist the temptation to push harder if the horse doesn't shift his weight. Just keep asking lightly until he shifts weight or steps over. Often the harder you push, the harder the horse pushes back (a good demonstration of how this principle works but without the desired result of the horse yielding to the slightest pressure).

Each time he shifts or moves in the direction you are asking, release and ask again. Soon, he will willingly be yielding, relaxing, and releasing to your touch because that is the path of least resistance for him.

This is how you ask for any movement from the horse while using these Techniques. Soon, if not already doing this, you will find yourself applying this principle to everything you do with your horse.

Note: *If the horse is resisting because there is an injury or excessive pain in an area while doing any Techniques that ask for movement, then he will continue resisting in order to protect the area. In any case, whenever you meet resistance, soften. If the horse still adamantly refuses to relax, he may need veterinary attention or time to heal.*

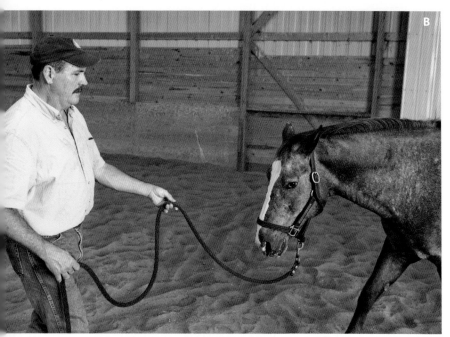

1.11 A & B Asking the horse to move forward with the slightest pressure (A). Releasing the pressure when the horse yields (B).

The Principle of Release of Tension in a Joint or Junction

Why, you may ask, is asking for movement in a relaxed state so important?

When you move a horse's joint or junction through a normal range of motion in a relaxed state, it releases tension in that joint or junction. You are staying under the survival response that wants to brace against or guard that tension or pain. When the horse moves through that in a relaxed state he lets go of the tension or pain.

When asking for movement properly and you find resistance in an area, it usually means there is tension or pain there. This resistance can be expressed by bracing against your touch, fidgeting, or walking away. This is how you know there is resistance, tension, or pain there. If you ask the horse to move through that resistance in a relaxed state, he will let go of the resistance.

Note: *Once you get used to this counter-intuitive way of reacting to the horse, you will experience the elation of discovering a completely new type of interaction with him. The results you see with this method will effortlessly increase and the new communication developed will spill over into other aspects of activity with your horse.*

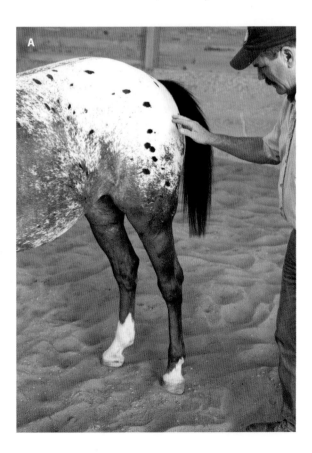
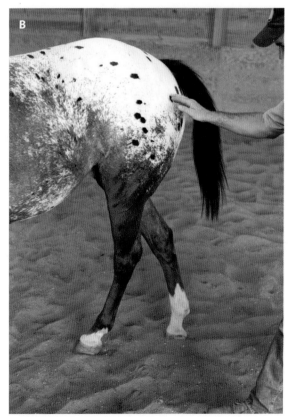

1.12 A & B Use the slightest pressure to ask the hind end to move to the side (A). Release the pressure when the weight shifts or the hind end moves (B).

CHAPTER 2

Working Environment and Safety

Experienced horse people know that the bond between human and horse can become very trusting over time. However, they are also aware that the horse is an instinctually programmed animal and can sometimes react to things we don't expect and at times when we least expect them!

As you may have guessed by now, we pay pretty close attention to the horse while using this method. You will soon find yourself better at reading the horse and anticipating some of these behaviors.

In handling the horse in general, the use of the principle of non-resistance alone can go a long way in preventing an undesirable situation from developing. By yielding, then immediately asking again, you help the horse's nervous system switch from "lead" mode to "follow" mode. Whenever you soften or yield to resistant (or even unpredictable) behavior, it is only to give the horse the opportunity to stop resisting, so that you can continue immediately to move ahead with what you were asking of the horse. It's not to let the horse do what he wants to do. Horses learn very quickly what works for them and what doesn't, and if you let go every time he resists, he'll resist whenever he wants you to let go. He'll be using the principle of non-resistance on you. You are there to help the horse. In order to keep both you and the horse safe, and to get this job done, you have to be the leader. This will go a long way toward keeping a situation safe.

The following five suggestions are based on my experience and are meant to keep both you and your horse safe and create an optimal working environment for a successful and enjoyable experience.

1. Where to Work

Ideally, I like to work on a horse in a stall. There are a number of reasons for this:

- I can step back from the horse to see what he has to say without him running off into the sunset.
- Stepping back and out of their immediate space makes many horses more comfortable, and they will release more readily. It gives the horse the room to move around (fidget) if he needs to while I continue working on him. In a sense, I am "yielding" to him as I continue my work.

- If I need the horse to stand still I can position him against the stall walls where I want him.
- If you are not familiar with the horse you are working on, you might like to have a way to exit the stall quickly if need be, such as leaving the door unlatched. This is up to your discretion. The nature of this work will in most cases keep the horse happy and "with" you.

2. Keeping a Connection with the Horse

When working on a new horse you may like to have another person nearby or holding the horse's lead rope. If you have an assistant in the stall, it is important that she stands back away from the horse and not interact with him in ways that will interfere with your ability to read his responses. This can include petting, rubbing ears, eyes or nose, or any other behavior your handler might find tempting. Your connection with the horse is what makes this work, and your ability to watch the horse's movement and responses to your touch is an important part of the work.

And no treats! Food is one thing that interferes with this process of "reading" and following the horse's responses and keeping him connected to you. So, be sure to remove food or any other distraction from the stall.

3. Using a Halter and Holding or Tying the Horse

I prefer not to hold or tie the horse unless the horse won't stay still for the work. If you do prefer to have someone hold or you tie him, it is impor-

tant that he is able to move his head and body as freely as possible without interfering with your ability to do your job.

If you decide to tie a horse you are unfamiliar with, or one that might be likely to pull back, then tie him in a way so that the rope will come loose easily, and not break the halter, hurt the horse, or disassemble the stall. Tie the lead rope to a piece of baling twine, or wrap it loosely around a bar or through the stall bars in such a way so it will pull free when tension is applied. This saves some time when trying to get a horse calmed down again after a pulling-back episode. If you are working alone and don't feel the need to tie the horse, you can drape the lead over the horse's neck as you are working. After time, you may become comfortable working on the horse without a lead rope. He is, after all, in a stall and can't wander too far.

Other tying tips:
- When going over the *Bladder Meridian* and *Ting Points* (see p. 24), you may want to tie or cross-tie a horse that will not stand or one that is "mouthy."
- When working on the *head, neck and shoulders* (see pp. 33 and 62) the horse needs to be able to move his head and front end freely so you may want to drape the lead rope over his neck, or have someone hold the lead loosely, while *not interacting* with the horse. By the time you have done the *Bladder Meridian Technique,* you probably have established a connection and communication with the horse that will have made him more comfortable with you—and you with him. You may tie the horse on a longer lead and still be able to do these exercises.

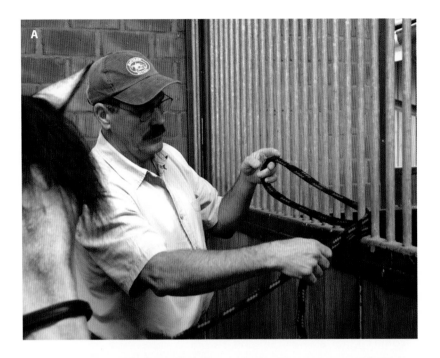

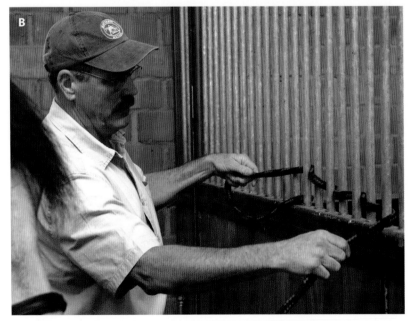

2.1 A & B By weaving the rope through the bars, if he pulls back, the rope will pull through (A). You can adjust the tension by weaving the lead rope through the bars, without tying (B).

■ When working on the hind end (see p. 104), the horse can again be tied with enough room to move his head freely.

Here is a safe method of tying in a stall with bars (figs. 2.1 A & B): By weaving the rope through the bars you can adjust the friction so that if he pulls a little bit the rope will not slip, but if he pulls back hard, the rope will pull through.

4. Techniques That Involve Handling the Hind Legs

It is important to be aware of the horse's state of mind, especially at first, until the horse is used to you. (Of course, this applies to the front end too, because a horse can act unpredictably at both ends! And always, keep an eye on the horse's ears whenever you first touch a horse that could be sore.)

This sense of awareness should become second nature in your handling of the horse; as it goes along with the sense of "feel" that you will be developing in the days to come. However, when starting out, it is important to be consciously aware of what you are doing and the effect you are having on the horse.

When you get to the hind end be aware the horse might be sore in the sacral area, gluteal muscles, hamstrings, groin, or abdominals, though since you will have already done the *Bladder Meridian Technique* (p. 24), you will have gone lightly over some of these areas, and his response then should have let you know if he has tension or pain there.

In fact, you may have already helped the horse to release some of this tension. However, you won't have covered the groin, abdomen, or between-the-legs areas, so it pays to be careful and keep an eye on his ears for signs of distress when *first touching* him anywhere he might be hurting.

The illustrations in Part Two show you how to best position your body in order to stay safe around the horse. When handling the legs be sure that the horse has room to move away from you rather than over you should something spook him. In my experience, 95 out of 100 horses would rather go around you if they have the option. It's best to leave a pathway to accommodate them.

Note: *This book includes many very effective Techniques for releasing tension in the hind end that do not involve handling the horse's hind legs. They should be used before exercises that involve handling the hind limbs, or any time you do not feel comfortable handling the hind limbs, and should become a regular part of your routine.*

5. Quiet Time and Frame of Mind

Pick a quiet time for your bodywork session. Feeding or anxious high traffic times in the barn will make your work less effective (and may wear you out). Assess your own frame of mind. Be as relaxed and calm as possible. Remember to breathe!

When you enter the stall, don't go straight for the horse's head. Stop for just a second and stand in a relaxed manner, maybe shift your weight from one leg to the other like a calm horse does, then walk (I like the word "amble") easily up to the horse's shoulder and let him know you're not there to jab him with a needle or something. Then ask him (using the principle of non-resistance) to step somewhere: maybe away from the wall to the center of the stall, or back away from you if he is pushing into your space—anywhere to get him to move his feet for you. Once you take the time to watch you'll notice that when you first ask him to do something, such as move his feet for you, and he yields and you soften, he will let out a sigh of relaxation, or lick and chew, or blink. Again, this gets his nervous system into the yielding or "following" mode, rather than the bracing or "leading" mode.

CHAPTER 3

How to Use This Book

When we started this project we had in mind a book that reflected this method of bodywork: something hands-on, easy-to-use, practical, and that would get results.

If you have read this far, you already have a good understanding of how the Masterson Method works and the principles of release involved. Now it is time to learn the individual Techniques that correspond to the three *key junctions* of the horse's body that most affect performance. Once you have done this, the book is designed to be taken into the stall with you to practice what you have learned.

Part Two

In Part Two, all the Masterson Method Techniques are presented and are divided into five practical sections. They start with *The Bladder Meridian Technique*. This first section sets the tone for your

work and your connection with the horse. In addition to being an effective way to release tension, this simple exercise is probably the most important in terms of experiencing and understanding how this interaction with the horse works.

The next sections (chapters 5–8) offer the Techniques. These exercises correspond to the *three key junctions* that most affect performance (see figs. 1.2 A & B, p. 5), as well as two very practical Techniques that help to release tension in the horse's back between the withers and the sacrum. Here is the complete list of what is included in Part Two:

1. *The Bladder Meridian Technique* (p. 24)
2. *The Poll-Atlas Junction:* occiput-atlas (p. 33)
3. *The Neck-Shoulders-Withers Junction:* cervical-thoracic C7-T1 (p. 62)
4. *The Hind-End Junction* sacroiliac-sacrolumbar T18-L1 (p. 104)
5. *The Back* (p. 143)

Each of these five sections in Part Two (chapters 2 to 8) describe several Techniques and includes:

- Anatomical descriptions and illustrations of the area.
- A step-by-step explanation how to perform the Technique.
- More detailed instructions.
- Practical tips.

- Notes on safety and working environment.
- Questions and answers covering issues that may arise.

Note: As different parts of the horse's body are interconnected, so certain Techniques in one area will contribute to releasing tension in other areas of the horse's body. These will be discussed in each chapter.

Part Three

Part Three puts the Techniques to good practical use. Chapter 9 lists 15 performance problems, explains their root causes, and suggests Techniques to use to resolve issues. Chapter 10 deals with issues specific to different breeds and disciplines of riding, and suggests Techniques to use before competition.

In practice you may not need to use all of the Techniques described for one area. Some will be better suited to you, and to your particular horse, than others. Think of them as different tools for your toolbox. General points to keep in mind:

- Understand the concept of *Search, Response, Stay, Release* (p. 11).
- Recognize the correlation between your touch and the horse's response. This is the *key* that opens the door.
- Be aware of the different levels of touch as you *use them.*
- Practice each chapter separately with this book at hand. Don't try to get it all at once but also look at this work as *a whole.*
- Look at the horse as a whole, too. It will make your work more effective.

- Keep going back to the basic principles introduced at the beginning of the book:

1. The horse's instinctive survival response is to *brace* against intrusion. If you can bypass this bracing response by softening, you can get the horse to release tension.

2. The horse is a herd animal and communicates through body language. It instinctively blocks pain and tension, and covers up weakness to survive. If you can read what's going on with the horse's body as you work you can get the horse to release that pain and tension.

3. The principle of non-resistance: Whenever you encounter resistance in the horse, if you soften or yield to that resistance it will allow the horse to release the pain or tension behind that resistance. When the horse is bracing against you, he can't release.

Reread the "Principle of Release of Tension in a Joint or Junction" (p. 15): When you move a horse's joint or junction through a normal range of motion in a relaxed state, it releases tension in that joint or junction. This is an extension of the principle of non-resistance: It's the *principle of non-resistance in motion* (if you want to get fancy about it).

4. If you understand these basic principles before you start your work, it will make the Techniques taught in this book very easy to learn, and will make the work more rewarding for both you and the horse.

5. Finally, this isn't really work! Have fun with it! In a very short time you'll be enjoying improved performance and a new level of communication and trust with your horse.

Where You Start Work

Symmetry and Asymmetry in the Horse

I find that most horses are the same as people in the sense that they are not perfectly symmetrical. A leg on one side may be a slight bit longer than the other, and one side or direction may be a little stronger or predominant just as most humans have a stronger or more predominant side. This initial asymmetry or imbalance may be emphasized with work and over time, and can eventually create larger imbalances that contribute to lameness.

Taking these differences into consideration, and from the perspective of what I find in working horses across many sports and disciplines, nine out of ten horses are naturally *right front-left hind* horses. This means they tend to favor, load or perform on the *right front-left hind diagonal*. They tend to be tighter behind the right side of the poll, generally a little stiffer in the right side of the neck, and get tighter in the left sacrum and hindquarter muscles. They often bend a little easier to the left and are more comfortable cantering on the left lead.

There are exceptions to every generalization: Some horses handle pain better than others and different horses compensate for discomfort or lameness by shifting loads back and forth to different areas. However, when muscle-tension patterns begin to develop in an asymmetrical way or unilaterally, loads are distributed unevenly and small issues can become problems.

So what does this have to do with where you start to work on a horse? When you begin, start at the front and on the side with the least tension. Releasing tension on the easier side first has the effect of releasing tension on the opposite side, and is much easier on the horse and you.

As explained earlier, the left front side is the easiest for most horses, so in the following sequence, work around the horse in a circle:

1. Left front
2. Right front
3. Right hind
4. Left hind

There are exceptions to this rule. If you find that your horse carries more tension or is more head-shy on the left side, start on his easier side, the right side.

Another notable exception is in the *Bladder Meridian Technique*. Here you start the same on the *left front* but instead go all the way to the *left hind Ting Point* before working on the horse's right side. All this is explained in detail in Part Two—coming up next.

Note: *While this book stands on its own, additional learning resources are available. See our website at www.mastersonmethod.com, and the resource section at the end of the book.*

PART TWO

Masterson Method™ Techniques

CONNECTION AND COMMUNICATION

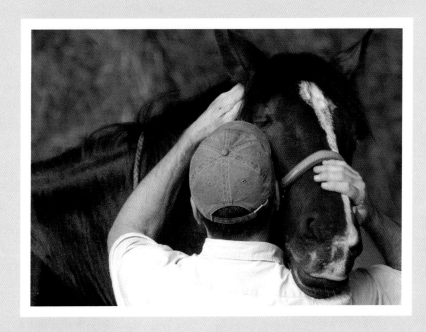

4

CHAPTER 4

The Bladder Meridian Technique

Before You Begin

GOAL: To bypass the horse's survival-defense response and connect directly with the part of the horse's nervous system that holds and releases tension.

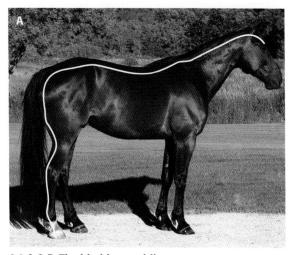

4.1 A & B The bladder meridian.

RESULT: This simple yet powerful Technique establishes the basis of communication between you and the horse through touch and response *(Search, Response, Stay, Release,* p. 11). It allows you to learn to "read" a particular horse and the horse to learn to "read" a particular human—you. It puts you both on the same page, so to speak, sets the tone for the interaction, and relaxes the horse and you.

As your first fact-finding tool, this Technique also shows you where the horse may be storing tension, and helps him to begin releasing it.

WHERE YOU WORK—ANATOMY

The *Bladder Meridian Technique* as we use it addresses the body and mind of the entire horse.

In Chinese medicine there are 12 primary acupuncture meridians in the body. The bladder meridian is one of the major acupuncture meridians in that it has a unique affect on balancing all of the others.

The bladder meridian runs along each side of the body parallel and just below the topline of the horse (figs. 4.1 A & B). It begins just behind the eye and runs over the poll between the poll and the ear, and from there continues down the neck about 2 to 3 inches below the crest, alongside the withers 2 to 3 inches beneath the topline, until it reaches the croup. From there it "leaves" the topline, going over the rump toward the "poverty groove"—the crease between the *biceps femoris* and *semitendinosus* muscles. Follow this groove down the hind leg, over the side of the hock just off the hind centerline of the leg, down the groove on the side of the cannon bone, over the fetlock, to its termination on the coronary band, as shown in the diagram (right).

RELEASING TENSION: THE EFFECTS

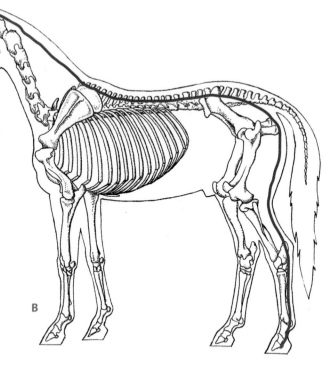

B

- The bladder meridian is a major acupuncture meridian to which all the other meridians connect, and it balances the entire meridian system.
- It runs over or near the main *junctions* of the horse on which you will work. Consequently, it serves as an initial "fact-finding" tool (showing horse sensitivity, for example) as well as getting first releases.
- It is easy to reach while allowing you to watch the horse's responses.
- It has a calming effect.
- However, the most important reason you begin the Masterson Method working on the bladder meridian is because it establishes the interaction of *touch and response* between you and the horse, at the same time as calming the horse and preparing him for the Techniques (bodywork) that follow.

You get a sense of how a particular horse is going to respond to your touch, and the horse gets an immediate sense of what he can expect from this interaction with you. The horse's nervous system learns to react to your touch in a way that

bypasses his *survival or defense response*. This will establish the basis of your communication with the particular horse you are working on. Along the way, the horse will let you know where he is "guarding" (i.e. blocking out) or bracing against the tension, and will begin to release that tension. The most valuable aspect of this Technique is the trust that develops between you and the horse as a result of this interaction.

Note: *If you practiced nothing else but the Bladder Meridian Technique on your horse—on a regular basis—it would make a noticeable difference in your horse's performance and behavior as a result. The Technique may seem "low energy" but, even alone, is effective in releasing tension in the horse's key junctions.*

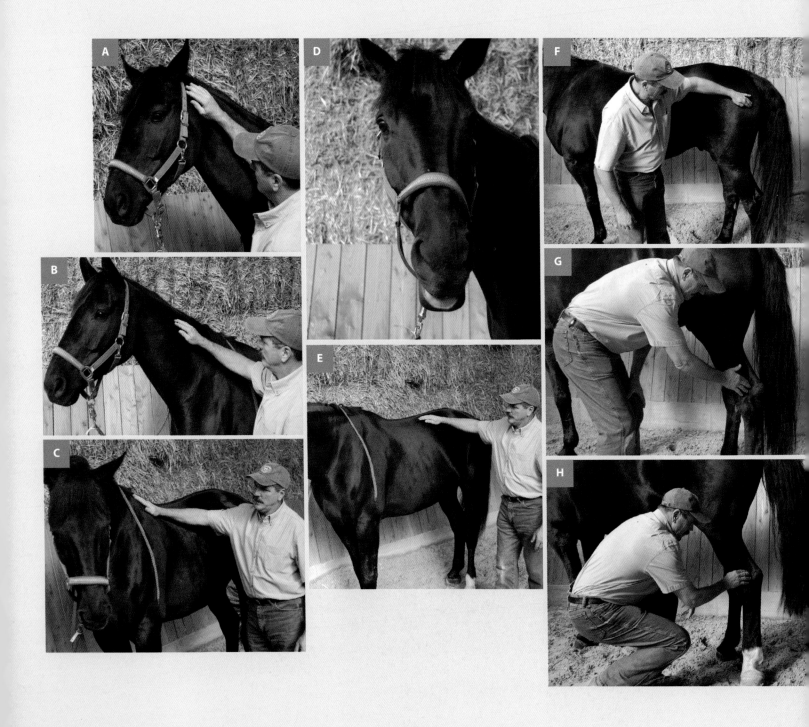

QUICK OVERVIEW: Step-by-Step

THE BLADDER MERIDIAN TECHNIQUE

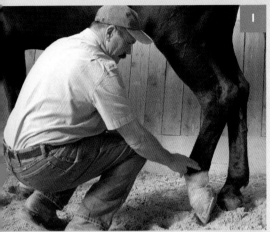

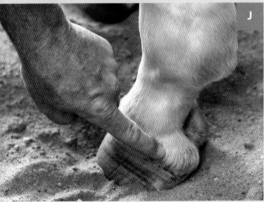

ONE: SEARCH

Step 1. Stand at the horse's head on the left side (A).

Step 2. Place the flat part of your fingertips, or cup the palm of your hand above the eye or on the poll just behind the left ear.

Step 3. Barely touching the surface of the skin, slowly (it should take about a minute to run your hand from the poll to the withers) run your hand down the bladder meridian (B).

TWO: RESPONSE

Step 4. As you move your hand and fingers down the meridian, watch closely for subtle signs or responses from the horse (C).

THREE: STAY

Step 5. Rest your hand and fingers over that spot, keeping your hand soft and the pressure light, waiting for a release. This may take one second, or one minute. Be patient. Breathe and relax…

FOUR: RELEASE

Step 6. … until you get a larger response of *Release*, in this case, licking and chewing (D).

Step 7. Then continue down the meridian, repeating these steps, along the back (E)…

Step 8. … over the rump (F)…

Step 9. …down the poverty groove (G)…

Step 10. …over the hock (H)…

Step 11. …over the pastern (I)…

Step 12. … and to the Ting Point—see sidebar, p. 29 (J).

Step 13. When you are finished, go to the right side and repeat.

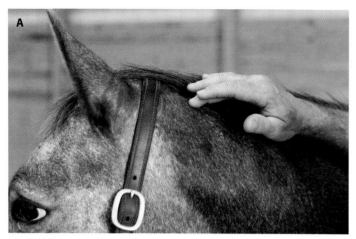

4.3 A **Using your fingertip.**

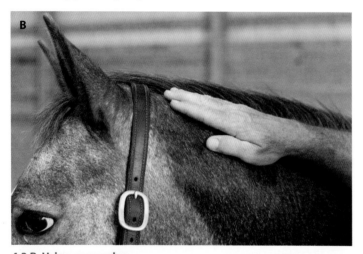

4.3 B **Using your palm.**

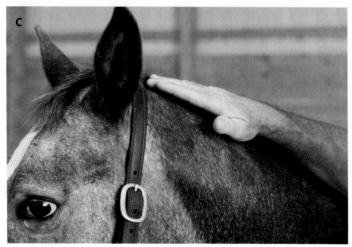

4.3 C **Using "air gap" pressure.**

Tips

Rule 1: Go softly: Use *air gap* pressure (non-pressure) barely touching the horse's hair or skin with your palm or the flats of your fingertips. Run them slowly along the meridian, watching the horse's responses to your touch—especially in the eye and lips (figs. 4.3 A–C).

Rule 2: Go slowly: Forget about the clock when doing this exercise. If you are anticipating or anxious, the horse will sense it. That doesn't mean he won't respond—he has to if you are going slowly enough and softly enough—but it will make your job easier if you are relaxed. Take a deep breath and move your hand very slowly along the meridian and watch for responses in his eyes and lips.

To give you an idea of how fast or slow you should be running your hand down the meridian, let's use the back of your hand, and the "one alfalfa, two alfalfa, three alfalfa" technique:

1. Hold your left hand in front of you with the back of your hand (knuckle side) facing you.
2. Place two fingertips of your right hand on your wrist.
3. Move your fingertips lightly (*air gap* pressure) from your wrist to the fingertips of your left hand.
4. Counting "one alfalfa, two alfalfa, three alfafa…" it should take six to eight flakes of alfalfa to get from your wrist to your fingertips. This is about the speed you should move your hand along the bladder meridian.

Ting Points

The termination of the meridians are called *Ting Points* in Chinese medicine. There are six Ting Points on each hoof and each is the termination point of a different meridian. Five of the six points are located around the coronary band, and one is located between the bulbs of the heel.

The Bladder Meridian Ting Point is on the outside where a "ridge" that runs down from the back quarter of the fetlock meets the coronary band.

Note: *The locations of acupressure points and meridians on the horse's body are not exact and differ with each body. This is only a general guide.*

As you aren't giving an actual acupressure treatment, don't worry that you may not be precisely on the bladder meridian. Follow the described path and let your intuition, and the horse guide you.

There are many books available on equine acupressure and Ting Points for those interested in learning more.

Ting Point Locations

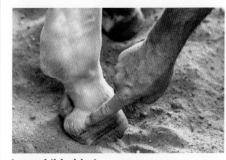
Lateral (bladder)

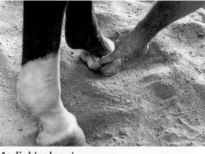
Medial (spleen)

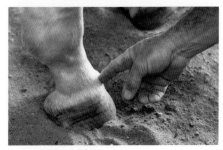
Front (stomach)

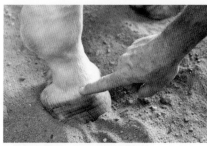
Quarter, lateral (gall bladder)

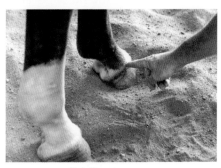
Quarter, medial (liver)

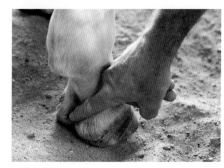
Behind (kidney)

When you get to the Ting Point that is the termination of the bladder meridian, stay there for a few seconds to see what kind of response the horse gives you. Sometimes you will get surprising releases from this—and the other Ting Points. A release doesn't necessarily mean that there is "tension" on that point, but rather it may be related to activity on the corresponding meridian.

You will start to notice, as you watch the horse's eyes, that there is a certain speed at which the horse stays connected to your fingers. Too fast, and you leave the horse behind; too slow, and the horse gets bored and stops "listening."

Rule 3: *Search, Response, Stay, Release.* When you get a response such as a blink or twitch of the lips, stop moving your hand and rest it there (still air gap pressure!) and wait for a larger, release response from the horse. The most common release will be licking and chewing, however, the horse may let out a sigh, or start to shift weight from leg to leg when he lets go. Once the horse shows this larger release response, move on.

More Suggestions

- Stop and hold your hand on a spot at any time if you sense that staying there may get a release.
- You can start over, or in a different place. You may switch hands, use both hands, stop and begin again, or retrace and go back over an area or spot. Don't worry: If you do this wrong your horse won't self-destruct or start to smoke.
- You may adjust the pressure or manipulate your fingertips or hand, or slow your hand down as you get responses.
- Make a mental note of all spots where your horse showed responses or releases. You will find that often, when touching on these partic-

ular areas or junctions again in the Techniques that follow, your horse will respond again in the same area and you might even find restrictions in movement that point to these areas.

Note: This exercise with its almost meditative qualities can become a regular part of your weekly routines. Soon your horse will start feeling "at home" so use it in various situations to "ground" him, such as when you have a quiet moment between showing, on the campground before or after a group trail ride, before a vet visit, or when trailering.

What Ifs?

- ### What if I get a response and stop, and then get no release?

First of all, be patient and allow the horse time to feel what is going on and time to be comfortable releasing. You are on the horse's agenda, not yours.

Secondly, keep your hand soft. If you feel nothing is happening, try softening your hand even more, or even taking your hand or fingertips off the hair. Watch the horse's eyes as you do this. You will see them soften. No matter how light you think your pressure is, lighten it even more.

The horse's first response when you find something will often be to try to block out what you are doing. But, if you stay long enough and lightly enough, the horse's nervous system will *have* to release tension.

If, after holding your hand over a spot for 30 or 40 seconds or so the horse doesn't respond, then move on. It doesn't mean you are doing it wrong, or that the horse is not cooperating. Be patient and move on slowly, possibly returning to the spot later.

■ *Sometimes I can't tell if the horse is blinking at something else, or at me.*

If you're not sure that the horse has blinked at a spot in response to your touch, move your finger back a few inches before that spot and slowly go over it again. If he blinks on the same spot, there is a correlation between what you're doing and what the horse is doing: It's a response. If not, move on.

Note: *Horses lick, chew, yawn, blink, and twitch all the time. With this exercise you are looking for the correlation between your touch and the horse's behavior or response to it.*

■ *What if my horse starts to fuss or walk away?*

Fidgeting is a sign that something is about to release. If your horse is standing quietly and you are waiting on a spot for a release and then he starts to fidget or take a step away, stay with him and continue what you were doing, but soften your hand just a little. Some horses will fidget more than others when they are about to release.

■ *What if he is "mouthy" or is constantly messing with the lead rope?*

Continue what you are doing and watch to see what happens. Often the horse will stop fussing after he releases a little bit, but some horses are just mouthy and fidgety. With a little practice,

you will get good at reading the releases and responses through the fussing. Sometimes the response you're looking for is when the horse *stops* fidgeting: Often, this is when he will release.

If you have a horse handler on the other end of the lead rope, the horse will often fuss with the handler. It's important that the handler does not interact with the horse while you're doing this Technique because it makes it difficult for you to "read" the horse.

■ *Can I tie the horse while doing this?*

Yes, especially if the horse is mouthy and won't leave you or the handler alone. I like to leave enough slack so that the horse can bend his neck or reach around a little bit. For safety, if you're in a stall, it's a good idea to tie the lead rope to a piece of baling twine or something that will break if the horse pulls back and starts to panic. The twine will break, the horse will calm down, and you'll all still be together in the stall—in one piece.

■ *What if my horse pulls his head away?*

First, give the horse a little room to pull away so that he doesn't feel trapped, but don't pull back on his head. If you soften the hand you're placing on the poll it will also help him to relax a little. If he still doesn't want your hand on his poll then start down the neck a little way until he is comfortable—and go from there. You can come back up to the poll after he has relaxed a little bit.

Take your time with head-shy horses. This is what they need the most. Most head-shy horses are this way because of pain or tension in the poll.

▪ How often should I do the Bladder Meridian Technique?

Do a little bit of this every day if your horse continues to respond. You don't need to do the whole meridian every time. If you do it too frequently and the horse stops responding, take a few days off and start up again later.

▪ If I'm not right on the meridian will it still work?

Don't worry about being exactly on the meridian. The horse will tell you where to work. You are learning to follow the horse's responses. The bladder meridian is an energy pathway and doesn't run in precisely the same place on every horse. You may, in fact, use this Technique anywhere on the horse's body, not just on the meridians.

▪ Will all horses respond and release the same?

After doing only a couple of horses you will notice that all horses are different. Depending on the horse and your individual sensitivity, the length of time you spend on the entire Bladder Meridian Technique will vary. Some horses are very stoic and take longer to respond and release. On these horses you have to go slower and pay very close attention to see the *subtlest responses*. Some show responses but won't release until you move past a spot, or step back away from them. Others start responding immediately (fig. 4.5).

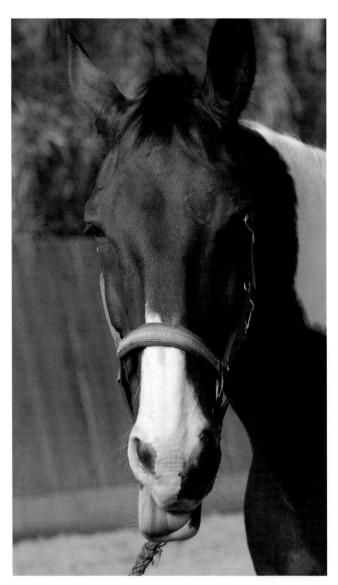

4.5 Not all horses respond the same. Some are stoic at first; others respond immediately.

CHAPTER 5

The Front End

Technique 1:
LATERAL CERVICAL FLEXION

Before You Begin

The *Poll-Atlas Junction* is arguably the most important of the three key junctions of the horse's body inasmuch as performance is affected.

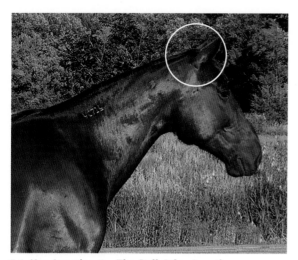

5.1 **Key Junction 1—The Poll-Atlas Junction.**

GOAL: To get lateral movement of the *poll, atlas and the rest of the vertebrae of the neck* by asking for movement in a relaxed state (see "The Principle of Release of Tension in a Joint or Junction," p. 15).

RESULT: Improved bending and suppleness in the poll and neck, and extension and suspension in the front end. As important: release of tension in the poll and atlas will release tension in the entire body.

WHERE YOU WORK—ANATOMY

Bones

Poll: For the purposes of this book I refer to the *poll* as the top of the horse's head (occiput).

Atlas: The vertebrae of the horse's neck are called the *cervical* vertebrae. The *atlas* is the first and most important cervical vertebra, behind the poll (fig. 5.2). It is also referred to as C1. To find the atlas, stand on the left side of the horse's neck and feel behind and to the side of the poll: You will feel and see a hollow space one inch behind the horse's jaw, and just behind that a bony bump or ridge. This ridge is the wing of the atlas (see fig. 6.2, p. 64).

Axis: The *axis* is the second cervical vertebra, or C2. From the atlas, slide your fingers a few inches farther down toward the direction of the shoulder and you will feel a flat area. The axis itself cannot ordinarily be felt, but it is located underneath this flat area.

Additional cervical vertebrae (C3, C4, C5, C6, and C7): The cervical vertebrae do not follow the top line of the neck, but run down the lower part of the neck (fig. 5.3). To find them, from the atlas run your fingers down along the *thickest* part of the neck. You will not feel the axis, but in a few inches you will feel a bump, which is the third vertebra, or *C3* then the fourth bump, *C4,* the fifth, *C5,* the sixth, *C6.* You will probably not feel the seventh, *C7,* because it is usually underneath the shoulder blade (scapula). If you cannot feel any of these bumps, find a skinnier horse to explore this part of the anatomy.

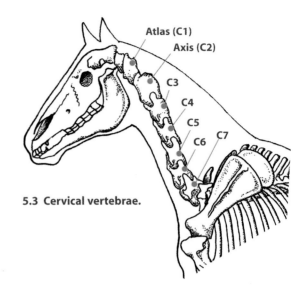

5.3 Cervical vertebrae.

You are working to release tension in the soft tissue interconnecting the poll, the cervical vertebrae, and major muscles that attach to these structures. Tension in these important muscles around the poll and atlas affect performance in other parts of the horse's body.

Muscles

Some of the major muscles attached to the neck and poll that affect movement and performance in other areas of the horse are:

Brachiocephalic (brachiocephalicus) or head-to-arm muscles, which are involved in moving the head from side to side, pulling the scapula forward, raising the scapula in collection, and bringing the foreleg forward (see fig. 6.2, p. 64).

Omotransverse (omotransversarius) muscles, which are also involved in raising the scapula and bringing the foreleg forward (again, see fig. 6.2, p. 64).

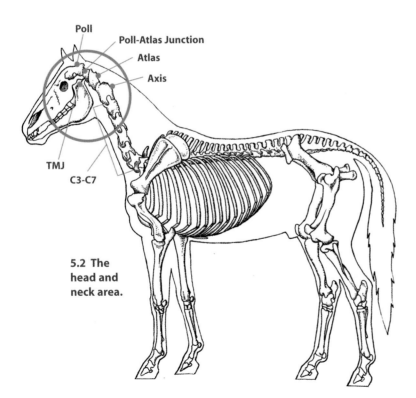

5.2 The head and neck area.

RELEASING TENSION: THE EFFECTS

Pain and tension anywhere in the horse's body is reflected in the poll. Conversely, when tension accumulates in the poll, things start going wrong in the rest of the body. Some examples:

■ Pain in the forelimb or foot can cause tension and pain through the muscles described on p. 34 into the neck and into the muscles of the poll and atlas. Excessive loading or pain in one forelimb can cause more tension and stiffness *on the same side of the neck,* and eventually resistance to bending in that direction. This can also cause pain and resistance to bending on the *same side in the area of the poll.* This can eventually lead to problems with the respective lead and lead changes, overloading the opposite front limb leading to soreness or lameness in that limb as well as the diagonal hind limb and restricted movement in the body overall. Conversely, when pain and tension accumulates in the poll, the *brachiocephalic* and other muscles connected to the forelimb tighten, thus taking away the ability of these and other muscles to absorb concussion. This puts more stress and strain on the forelimb and foot, which can then lead to injury or lameness, causing more pain in the poll, and so on: a vicious cycle.

5.4 The nuchal and supraspinaous ligament connection.

■ Pain in the saddle area or back can create tension in the area of the top of the poll. Tension through the muscles of the back and top line along the *supraspinous* and *nuchal ligaments* contract the back and create tension and pain in the poll (fig. 5.4). The same vicious cycle of pain and tension affects the poll and back.

■ The *atlas* and *sacrum* (see fig. 7.2 A, p.105) are connected. When there is tension on the atlas, there will almost always be tension on the sacrum, and vice versa: tension on the sacrum means tension on the atlas. That's just the way it is. When you release tension on the atlas, you are also releasing tension on the sacrum, and when you work on the sacrum, you are also working on the atlas. How cool is that?

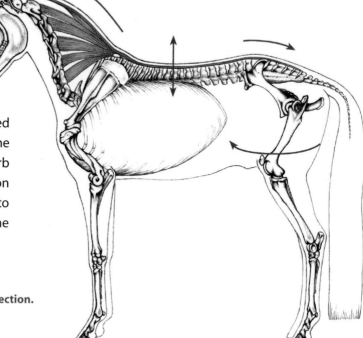

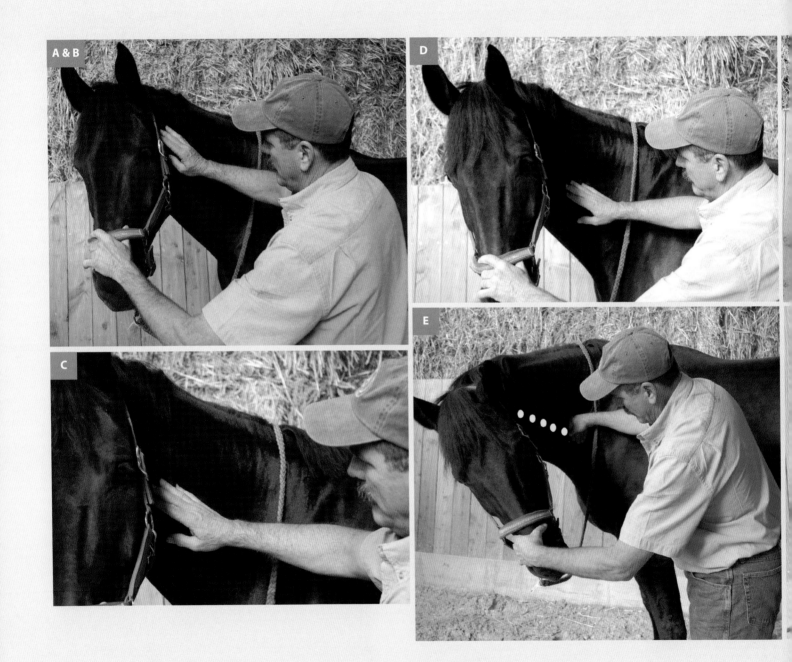

QUICK OVERVIEW: Step-by-Step

TECHNIQUE 1: LATERAL CERVICAL FLEXION

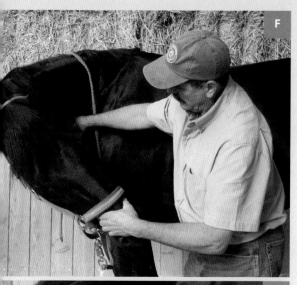

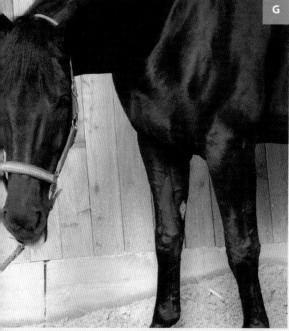

Step 1. Place your *left* hand on the horse's nose. Place your *right* hand or fingertips on the bottom of the wing of the atlas about 4 inches below and behind the ear (A). Your fingers should be on the bony part of the atlas, not in the groove between the jaw and the atlas.

Step 2. Bring the nose slightly toward you with the *left* hand. Put *very gentle* pressure toward the opposite ear with the fingertips or palm of your *right* hand.

Watch for the eye to soften, feeling for relaxation in the atlas and poll. You are asking the horse to relax the muscles of the atlas and poll (B).

Step 3. Soften both hands. Move your *right* hand 2 or 3 inches down the vertebrae of the neck, keeping your *left* hand on the nose (C).

Step 4. Bring the nose back farther, resting the fingertips of the *right* hand on the neck. Wiggle the nose gently, watching for the eye to soften (D).

Soften both hands again and move the *right* hand further down the vertebrae of the neck. Step back toward the shoulder as you go.

Step 5. Bring the nose back farther, resting the fingertips of the *right* hand farther down on the neck, stepping back as you go to make room for you to bring his head closer to the shoulder (E). Wiggle the nose gently, watching for the eye to soften.

Soften both hands again and move the *right* hand farther down to the lower neck.

Step 6. Keep bringing the nose back farther toward the point of the shoulder, stepping back as you go (F). Wiggle the nose as you focus the bending of the lower neck with your right hand.

Step 7. Step back and allow the horse to release: lick and chew, yawn, sneeze, snort, or "shake loose" (G).

Technique 1 in More Detail

After the *Bladder Meridian Technique*, the *Lateral Cervical Flexion Technique* is the first step toward releasing tension in the poll and atlas and asking for movement in this area. Starting on the left side:

1. Start by resting your left hand softly on the horse's nose.
This "nose hand" is the hand you will use to ask for movement (fig. 5.5).

2. Position your "neck hand."
Then place your palm or the flat of your fingertips of your right hand (the "neck hand") below and behind the wing of the atlas (about 3 or 4 inches below and behind the ear). Use very, very light pressure *(egg yolk)* here. The right hand should not be a pushing point, but a kind of fulcrum around which you are asking the horse to bend and move in a relaxed state (fig. 5.6).

3. Ask for movement.
Keeping the left hand softly on the nose, gently ask him to bring his head toward you. When you feel him soften toward you, give his nose a slight wiggle.

Then, keeping his nose in this position with your nose hand, soften both hands, take a small step back toward the horse's shoulder, slide your right hand a few inches farther down the vertebrae of the neck, and again ask him to bring his nose a little farther back toward you, giving the nose a little wiggle. Repeat this on down the horse's neck, stepping back and bringing his head back a little farther each step of the way.

Nose back, wiggle, soften, step back.
Nose back, wiggle, soften, step back.
Nose back, wiggle, soften, step back. Easy!

Tips

- Don't worry too much about the exact placement of your hand. As long as the horse is moving the muscles and vertebrae of the neck through his natural range of motion in a general way, you are doing it correctly.

    However, one horse will not give you the same range of motion as another (see p. 39).

    Except with very stiff or old horses, by the time you have worked your right hand all the way down his neck, the "nose-hand" should have guided the horse's nose to a point in the area of his shoulder.

- Get the horse to work *with* you. You are circumventing the horse's flight or fight instinct by giving him nothing to brace against. Gently asking the horse to bring any part of the body voluntarily to you will be much more effective than forcefully initiating movement. Asking him to volunteer puts the horse mentally *with* you, and his nervous system automatically in the "release" mode, rather than the resist or "survival" mode.

    The way to get the horse to move with you—meaning to yield to your touch—is for you to *soften* when you run into resistance. *Show him that the path of least resistance is to move with you, not against you.* We humans tend to push, hold, or pull when the horse resists what we are asking. We need to resist this instinct and—

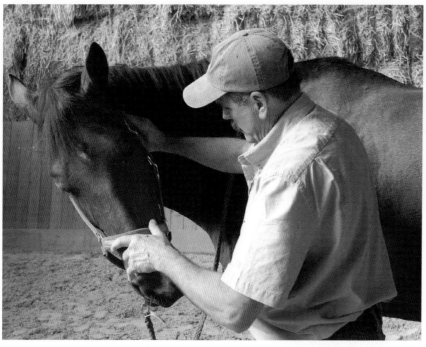

5.5   **Ask for gentle movement (wiggle, wiggle) with the "nose hand."**

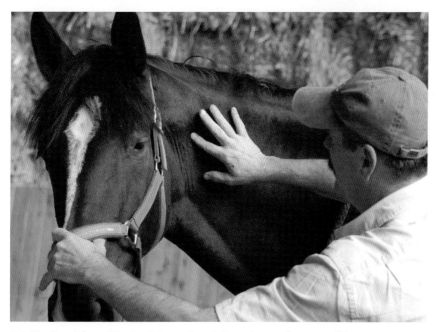

5.6   **The "neck hand" is the fulcrum hand. Keep it as soft as possible.**

REMINDER
The Main Principles of Release

These principles apply during the *Lateral Cervical Flexion* exercise and in every other Technique that involves movement.

When you move a horse's joint—or junction—through its natural range of motion in a relaxed state, tension is released in that joint or junction.

This is how you use the Masterson Method to bypass the horse's *survival or bracing response* and allow the horse to release tension in key joints and junctions of the body that most affect performance:

1. By staying under his *survival or bracing response,* you can move the joint or junction *in a relaxed state.*

2. By giving the horse *nothing to resist,* you stay *under his survival or bracing response.*

3. By staying *soft and slow enough,* you give him *nothing to resist.*

4. By following *the horse's responses* to your touch, you are able to stay *soft and slow enough,* which allows you to *bypass the horse's survival or bracing response.*

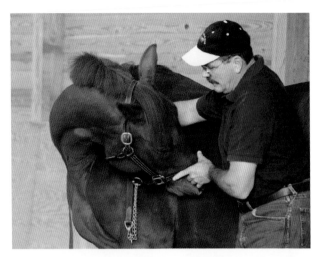

5.7 Ask for movement in a relaxed state.

even though it may seem counterintuitive—release pressure instead. This way you get both the horse's mind and nervous system to work *with* you instead of bracing *against* you.

Note: *Avoid "clawing" the horse's nose, especially with fingernails. Keep your nose-hand soft and use the flat of your fingers.*

- Do a little on one side, and then the other. It's good to alternate side to side if you need to go over an area more than twice in a row. If you go over one area over and over, the horse will start just "going through the motions" rather than releasing. Go back and forth, from side to side. You can tell enough is enough when the horse stops giving you releases.

- Step back and look for signs of release. This is the fun part! Allow the horse to "shake loose" or give any other signs of release such as yawning, licking and chewing, blinking, shifting weight from side to side. When you're not getting the releases you think you should be getting, step back into the corner, and give him a chance to let go (fig. 5.8).

Note: *When you step back to see what the horse has to say, step WAY back. Some horses need a lot of space between you before they're comfortable enough to show you the signs of release. We may think that by not touching them we are giving them enough room, but they're thinking "Get OUT of my SPACE, MAN!" in a silent, horse-sort-of way.*

REMINDER
Important! Don't force it!

Some horses are more flexible than others. One horse may find it easy to bend the neck and follow your nose-hand, while another might be physically unable to reach around even half-way. Resistance may be caused by stiffness or lack of range of motion, or by soreness. In either case, go softly and don't force it. Your goal is to release tension in the soft tissues around the vertebrae by asking them to move *in a relaxed state* (fig. 5.7). If you find yourself bracing against the horse, it isn't working. Soften!

You are only looking for an incremental *improvement in range of movement* each step of the way, not to try to get the horse to bend or flex beyond where he can comfortably go. Some horses are naturally stiffer than others, especially as they get older. If you get an improvement or release response each step of the way as you go along you will get results without the risk of harming the horse. You can then go over the area again, getting improvement.

Each time you go over an area and obtain releases, it's as if you are "peeling layers of an onion."

What Ifs?

■ **What if the horse doesn't think it's so easy? What if the horse resists?**

In general when a horse pulls away, your first impulse is to pull back. Here's a little tip: Don't pull back! Yield with the asking hand slightly, just enough so that he stops pulling, then immediately ask again. If you give the horse nothing to resist against, even for just a split second, he'll usually stop resisting. You can ask him to keep his head in the general area until he relaxes, but when he stops fussing, you must immediately soften your hand before asking again. By doing this, you'll find yourself giving the horse a little room to resist and then relax while keeping his nose "in the neighborhood."

When the horse pulls his head away, it's almost always for a good reason, usually because of pain or tension in the poll. By softening, you're giving him a chance to release the tension.

■ **What if the horse tries to get his nose out from under my hand?**

Some horses just do not like your hand on their nose. When this happens, you can either use the halter's noseband instead of his nose, or hook your thumb under and your index finger over the noseband while keeping your hand on the nose. This way, when he tries to shake you off you are able to keep your hand on his nose without having to grab (fig. 5.9). But remember to keep your hand as soft as possible when "wiggling" the nose.

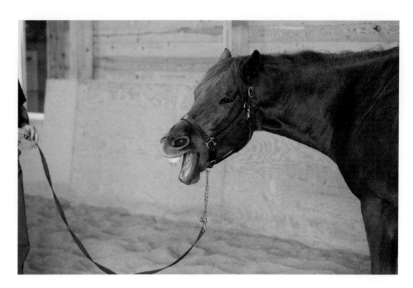

5.8 Step way back, and give the horse a chance to release.

Note: *You can be firm with the horse when asking him to do what you want—BUT you have to remember to soften your hand immediately when he yields to you or he will continue bracing. If you find yourself bracing with the horse, it isn't working. Remember the principle of non-resistance.*

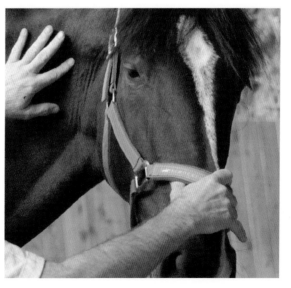

5.9 Slip your thumb under the noseband, and your index finger over the top.

■ *What if he pushes his nose around to his shoulder immediately?*

The horse is bracing by anticipating what you'd like him to do and "performing" the task ahead rather than staying with you. Ask him to bring his nose back out to the front, relax there, and then ask for movement again.

■ *What if he "corkscrews" his head sideways, or "flattens his head" as I bring the nose around?*

The horse will "corkscrew" his neck and flatten his head sideways if the vertebrae of the upper neck are not able to flex laterally. What is happening is he is trying to do what you are asking (bring his nose to the side) but since the vertebrae of the upper neck are not moving laterally, he does it by flexing his upper neck dorsally (i.e. bringing his chin downward) and bending his lower neck laterally, which puts his head on a sideways plane. It looks like he's "corkscrewing" his neck.

You can help him release some of this lateral restriction in the upper neck by gently lifting upward on the nose as you bring the head around. Lift a little and soften a little… lift a little, and soften a little. Remember not to force it. You are just looking for an improvement.

■ *What if he throws his head and absolutely refuses to relax?*

When this happens it may be an indicator that there is a lot of discomfort in this area. You are now bringing the horse's attention to it and any contact at all is too much. When he absolutely won't soften, move to an area of his body that is more comfortable and work your way back to the poll. Try starting on the opposite side or, if that is too reactive, at the lower neck, working your way gradually up the neck to the atlas. If this doesn't work, hold the palm of your hand an inch away from the poll and soon he will stop throwing his head and start to release. You don't even need to touch him. In most cases it won't take a horse long to realize that you aren't hurting him and he will start releasing. From there you may gradually be able to use *air gap* or *egg yolk,* if you need it.

Note: *The most common mistake in this exercise is to use too much pressure with the hand on the neck. If this is where the horse is sore, he will brace against it or resist, either internally or outwardly. Keep the neck hand as soft as possible as you wiggle the nose.*

Soften the hands even more until you see the eyes soften, or blink. When he blinks or his eyes soften, then you are soft enough.

He may also become uncomfortable and start to throw his head if you spend too much time doing the Technique without giving him a chance to release. Remember to step back from time to time to see what he has to say. When you do step back, give him at least 30 seconds—or more if you think he needs it—before continuing.

■ *What if my horse walks forward or keeps moving his hind end away from me to keep from bending in the neck?*

Some horses do this to try to avoid bending in the neck. Some try to walk forward, others simply

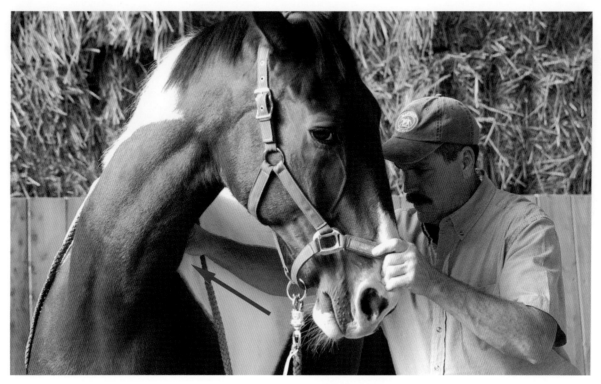

move their rump around in a circle until you get dizzy and quit.

The first thing to do: When in doubt, soften the hands. Try to "stay under the radar" by keeping the horse relaxed, but still get the movement you want.

If the horse still walks forward or moves his hind end away, every time he moves his feet, use your body weight to ask him to step away from you (move laterally) each step he takes (fig. 5.10). This will do three things:

1. It keeps him from spinning around you.
2. It will eventually have him standing against the side of the stall, where he can't spin around.
3. When the horse moves laterally, he tends to let go of any bracing.

■ *What if the horse fidgets?*

If the horse fidgets or fusses in any way, consciously soften your touch but do not take your hands off. Soften and relax the pressure, then immediately ask again. *Fidgeting is a sign that the horse is about to release.* When you soften, it gives the horse a chance to release.

■ *Why does the horse fidget?*

If you are doing the exercise properly, meaning softly and under the horse's radar, then the fidgeting comes when he is feeling some tension about to release. This bothers him just a little bit and he fidgets as he lets it go. In this case, the solution is

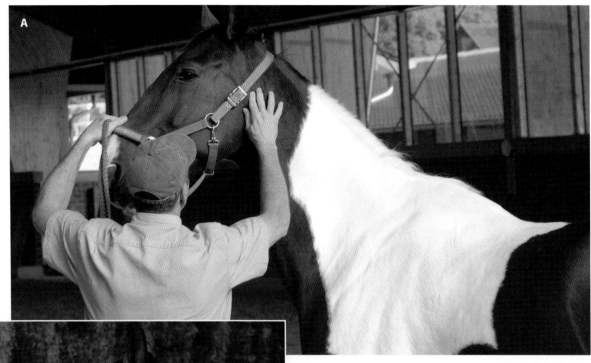

5.11 A & B If the horse braces, raises his head, or fidgets, then soften your hands and yield, just "keeping him in the neighborhood."

with it just a little longer helps him to let it go.

The horse will also fidget if the pressure you are using is too much and you are bringing his attention to the tension in an uncomfortable or even painful way. In this case, the solution is also to soften your hands and wait for him to relax. Then you continue what you are doing, asking for movement in a relaxed state. When his eyes are soft or blinking, you are soft enough. If you feel even the slightest bracing, it will be difficult for him to release.

In either case, the solution is to soften your hands so that the horse softens, and then continue gently with the movement (figs. 5.11 A & B).

to soften your hands slightly and ask the horse to stay with the exercise for just a second longer. Then step back and see what he has to say. Often, staying

Technique 2: HEAD DOWN

Before You Begin

GOAL: To release tension in shortened muscles behind the poll by positioning the horse's head down.

RESULT: Improved suppleness in the poll, and release of tension in the entire body.

WHERE YOU WORK—ANATOMY

You are already familiar with the *poll,* and *cervical (neck) vertebrae.* With this *Head Down Technique* you are working directly on muscles, large and small, that attach to the poll, atlas, and other vertebrae of the upper neck. Many of these muscles work to rise up, hold and turn the head and upper neck.

You will also be working on muscles and ligaments that connect to the withers, sternum, and foreleg. An important part is the *nuchal ligament.* It is the main component of the "suspension bridge" that runs from the poll, over the top of the withers, down the top of the spinal column via the *supraspinous ligament,* to connect to the sacrum (see fig. 5.4, p. 35).

RELEASING TENSION: THE EFFECTS

The poll accumulates a great deal of stress and tension that the horse is unable to release on his own. In addition to mechanical stress that is exerted on muscles of the poll and atlas through movements of the head and neck, *mental stress*—worry and fear—also greatly affects the poll and atlas. Pain anywhere in the body will also result in stress and tension in the poll and atlas. I have found that pain in the front feet, and pain in the back can contribute greatly to tension in the poll and atlas.

When you begin to pay close attention to what the horse is telling you, you will see that when tension in the poll and atlas is released, tension in the neck, shoulders, and hind end—especially in the gluteals, hamstrings and sacrum—relaxes as well.

Technique 2 in More Detail

A horse with a lot of tension may initially not want to lower his head. In addition, some horses instinctively feel very vulnerable in this position. Due to this fear factor it may be difficult to get him to lower his head. If this is the case you may choose to move on to the next Technique, which accomplishes the same goal. Don't feel that you have to do every Technique on every horse. Different Techniques work in different situations. Consider them as tools in your toolbox.

QUICK OVERVIEW: Step-by-Step

TECHNIQUE 2: HEAD DOWN

Begin by relaxing the muscles of the poll and atlas as much as possible with the *Lateral Cervical Flexion Technique* (p. 33).

Step 1. Stand on the left side of the horse's neck, facing the neck. Place your *left* hand on the forehead and your *right* hand just behind the poll (A).

Step 2. With both hands, gently ask the horse to lower his head. Every time he yields to your pressure, yield to his and immediately ask for more. When he raises his head, don't use force; just gently ask him to lower it again (B).

Step 3. With the *right* hand, massage the muscles behind the poll. Start with *grape* pressure gradually increasing to *lemon* pressure if the horse stays relaxed with it. You can use the *left* hand to gently ask the horse to keep his head down as you massage with the right (C).

When the muscles relax as you massage, get into a rhythm that gets the horse's head bob-bing up and down loosely. This moves this key junction through a range of motion in a relaxed state as you massage.

Step 4. Step back and allow the horse to shake loose, let it out, and show signs of release (D).

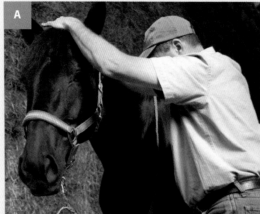

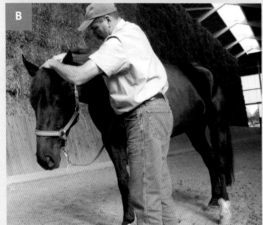

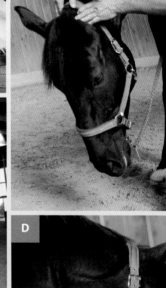

Convincing the horse to lower his head should be a gentle but consistent process.

1. Position yourself.

Stand on the left side of the horse and place the palm of your right hand gently just behind the crest of the poll. Place your left hand on the poll as shown (see fig. 5.12 A).

2. Ask, yield, ask.

Slowly apply gentle pressure to ask the horse to bring his head down (see fig. 5.12 B). The moment he yields the slightest bit, *relax the pressure for a split second* without removing your hand, then immediately ask again, releasing pressure each time as a response to the slightest yielding on the horse's part (fig. 5.13). Keep your hands soft. You can be *firm* without being hard with your hands. The horse can sense any tension in your hands.

3. Massage gently.

Once the horse has lowered his head to the point where you feel the muscles begin to soften, keep your left hand on the poll to let him know you want him to stay down while using the palm of the right hand to gently massage behind the poll (fig. 5.14). If you sense the horse is tensing up, lighten your touch and continue. You may have to do this in small steps; ask him to lower a bit, massage for a moment, then ask some more.

Use the *flat* of your fingertips to massage, not the points of your fingertips. "Clawing" into the

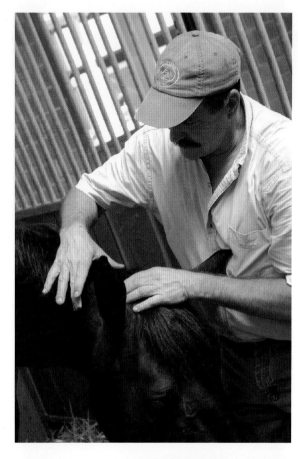

5.13 Head Down: Ask, soften immediately when he yields, then ask again.

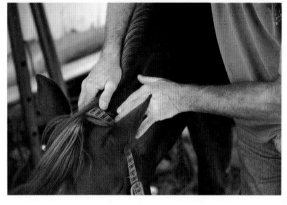

5.14 Massage the muscles just behind the poll, under the headstall.

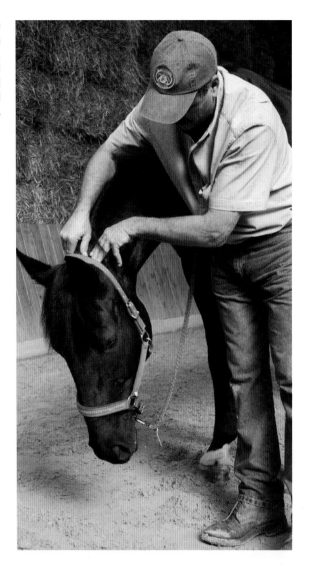

horse will instinctively cause him to tense. The softer and slower you begin, the better your results.

4. Massage deeply.

Once the horse is relaxed, you can massage with *lemon* or even *lime* pressure, as long as he stays relaxed. When the surface muscles relax, feel for smaller, harder knots underneath (fig. 5.15).

Massage directly on the harder knots a little longer. You may not be able to completely remove the knot, but it may shrink in size. This depends on how long the knot has been there and what might be causing it. You will find that all horses are different in this respect.

Once the horse has relaxed a little and become used to this, you can bob his head as you massage. This moves the *Poll-Atlas Junction* through little ranges of motion in a relaxed state, releasing even more tension as you massage.

Ideally, work until the horse's eyes are soft or closed and his head is bobbing as you massage. There is no set amount of time to do this. This can be a successful exercise, whether it lasts two seconds, two minutes or ten minutes. If you are not sure, you can step back at any time and see what the horse has to say, and then continue again if you think you could do more.

5. Step back and let the horse feel the release.

You will be surprised how much tension some horses have in this area and how much just a little work there will release it. You will start to get a feel for this as you practice more.

Tips

- Asking the horse to lower his head will result in shortening and softening of the muscles behind the poll and on top of the atlas. When the horse's head is down, his nose is extended in a relaxed position and these muscles relax, enabling you to massage effectively directly on the muscles. Three points to remember:

1. The best way to get the horse to relax these muscles is to get him to lower his nose to the ground.

2. The best way to get the horse to lower his head is to ask him.

3. You can't win a wrestling match with a horse, so you'd better learn how to ask him properly. The key to successfully asking the horse to lower his head is in the timing. This is something that may take some practice for you, and may involve some training for your horse.

Safety Notes: *Keep your head off to the side when you are massaging with the head down (fig. 5.16). The horse can come up faster than you can get out of the way.*

Don't move your feet suddenly with the horse's head down. It often startles the horse so it comes up again. If you bend your knees and shift your weight a little bit before moving your feet, the horse won't startle. This also works any time you are around or approaching a nervous horse. The horse will notice this and will stay relaxed. Notice how this works with horses standing around the paddock or pasture in a group. If one horse picks up a foot quickly, the others will often react by tensing or jerking. When a horse shifts his weight slowly before picking up the foot, the others don't react.

- Remember to breathe. The horse will sense this and relax.

- Throw away the clock! If you are in a hurry, it won't work!

- Be prepared to do this exercise a few times until

you and the horse are used to it. The *Head Down Technique*—with you on top—puts him in a very vulnerable position, so don't get angry with him for instinctively protecting himself.

- Sometimes we become so focused on the task at hand that we don't notice when the horse needs a break. Step back now and then to see what he has to say. You can always start again where you left off. Stay mindful of the horse!

What Ifs?

- ***What if the horse resists?***

There are three things you can do to get the horse to yield to your pressure:

1. Use the *Lateral Cervical Flexion Technique* to lead into *Head Down*. Bring his head to the side then slowly ask him to lower his head from

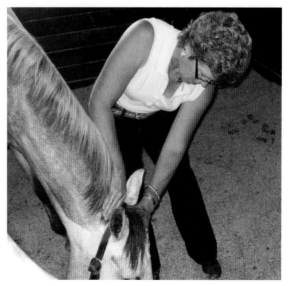

5.16 Keep your head off to the side.

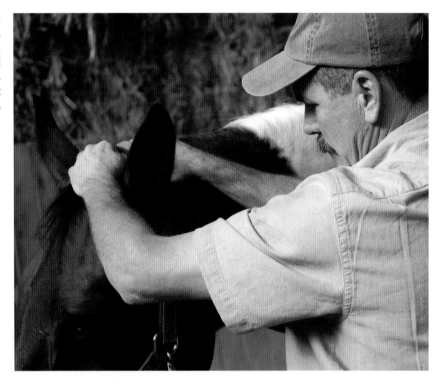

5.17 If he will only lower his head half way, stop asking and start massaging. Often, he'll relax and go lower.

What if he will only lower his head to a certain point and then stops?

Start gently massaging the neck where he stops lowering. Often he will relax even more after a minute. Sometimes gently rocking the neck will help. Keep your left hand gently on the poll to let him know you want him to keep his head where it is (fig. 5.17).

What if he lowers to a certain point, then throws his head up again?

If he forcefully throws his head up, do not try to hold his head down by force. Instead, *keep your hands loosely on his poll or neck as he brings his head up* then immediately begin asking him to come down again. If you allow him to stay up he will quickly learn to raise his head.

Sometimes you can prevent him from starting to bring his head up. If you sense that he is tensing or is ready to bring his head up, soften your hand first, and he may well relax. When you stop forcing him to stay down before he even tries to come up, he will stop forcing. Then you can begin asking again.

there. Lateral movement helps to ease the bracing response and rest the horse's mind.

2. Apply gentle pressure and release it slightly for just a moment, not waiting for the horse to yield. You may feel the horse let go a little bit as you release. This will often get the process started. Then, immediately ask again.

3. Use your left hand to create a "glass ceiling" that you want him to stay below each time he lowers his head more. When his head comes up against your hand, it gives him something to bump against. When he goes down, away from your hand, release pressure.

Technique 3:
HEAD UP

Before You Begin

GOAL: To shorten and soften the muscles of the poll, atlas, and neck as with the *Head Down Technique,* and also to allow movement of the poll, atlas, and neck in a relaxed state by resting the horse's head in an *up* position (see "The Principle of Release of Tension in a Joint or Junction in a Relaxed State," p. 15).

RESULT: Improved suppleness in the poll and release of tension in the entire anatomy. This Technique is also integral to releasing tension in the sacrum and major muscles of the hind end.

WHERE YOU WORK—ANATOMY

As with *Head Down, you* are releasing tension in the muscles and connective tissue of the poll, atlas, and neck.

This Technique is also very effective in releasing tension found in many dressage horses in the throat latch area and jaw. It also affects muscles that connect the head and neck to the forearm, shoulder, and scapula.

RELEASING TENSION: THE EFFECTS

When you move the head and joints of the neck through a range of movement in a relaxed state, you release tension in the muscles above, as well as the muscles that attach here, such as the *brachiocephalicus, omotransversarius, sternomandibular* muscles that affect the forelimbs (see fig. 6.2, p. 64).

Releasing tension in this junction of the poll and atlas also has a profound effect on releasing tension on the sacrum and in major muscles of the *hind end.*

From a neuromuscular and biomechanical viewpoint, the atlas and the sacrum are the two opposite ends of the same spinal column that is the primary nerve-distribution channel through the horse's body. The muscles that these nerves control and the skeleton they are attached to enable all of the horse's components to work together in a coordinated manner. Tension accumulated in one area affects another area.

On a practical level this connection will become apparent once you start noticing release responses the horse gives you in the *hind end* while you are working on the *poll,* such as wobbling behind, or dropping one hip and then the other. Occasionally, a horse will kick out or snap a hind foot up simultaneously as he's giving you a release response on the front end. This can especially be seen in horses with extreme tension and pain in the hamstrings.

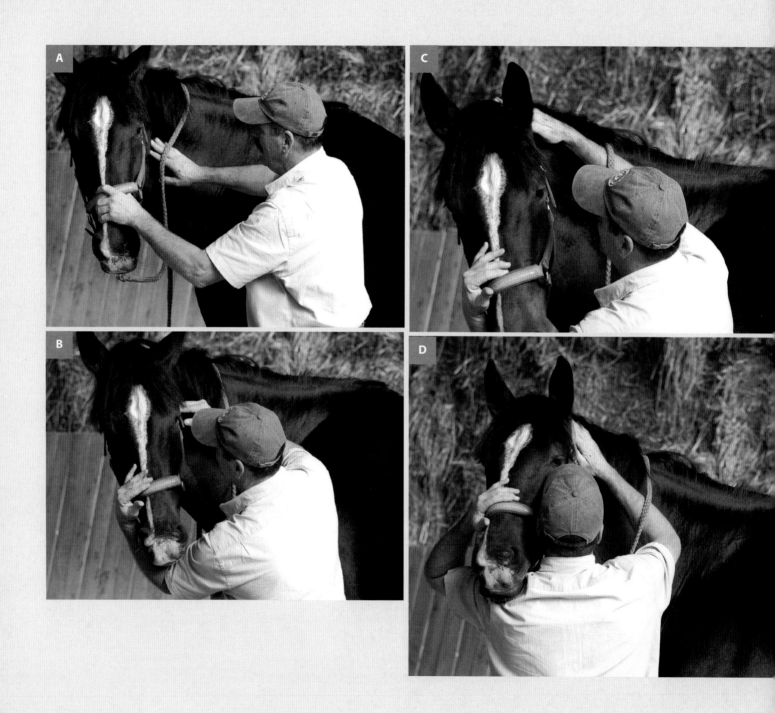

QUICK OVERVIEW: Step-by-Step

TECHNIQUE 3: HEAD UP

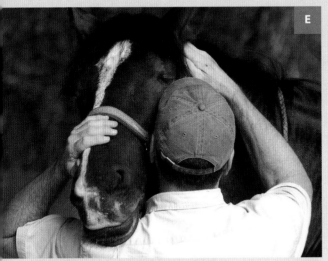

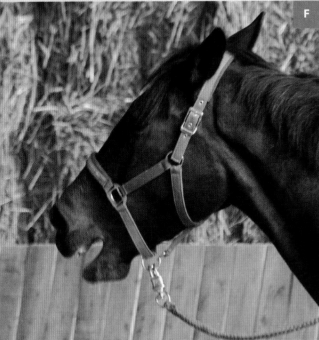

Step 1. Bring the horse's nose to the side until he is relaxed, as described in *Technique 1: Lateral Cervical Flexion* on p. 33 (A).

Step 2. Keeping the fingers of your *left* hand on the nose, pivot your elbow of the same arm down under the jaw and gently lift so that the weight of the horse's head rests on your arm (B).

Step 3. Slide your *right* hand on top of the *atlas,* and gently massage the muscles above the atlas on this side (C).

Step 4. Slide the horse's head up onto your shoulder (D). If he tenses, continue support-ing his head on your arm with one hand on the nose and the other on top of the neck or atlas.

Step 5. Use the *Search, Response, Stay, Release* Tech-nique to find responses around the poll. Watch the eyes for responses. Stay soft with your fingers.

Step 6. Massage the muscles behind, below, and around the poll, and ask for gentle range of motion in this junction (E).

Step 7. Step back and allow the horse to shake loose and release (F).

These correlations are what you are looking for that enable the horse to tell you in real time what is going on with his body. This Technique is one of the most effective and rewarding exercises you can do for your horse (and you).

Technique 3 in More Detail

In the last section, I gave you some advice for the *Head Down Technique:* "One of the best ways to get the horse to relax muscles is to get him to lower his nose to the ground." Here is the other way of doing this: the *Head Up Technique.* Your goal is to take the weight of the head and neck off his poll and atlas by resting his head on your arm or shoulder (fig. 5.19).

Once his head is there, the muscles and connective tissue that put tension on the poll and atlas can relax. Simply by being in this relaxed position, the horse is able to let go of deep-seated tension he is rarely able to let go on his own.

You may have to use small steps to get the feel for this Technique and to get the horse used to it. It's important to go slowly, stay as relaxed as possible, and give the horse time to relax into this

position before actually "doing" anything. Eventually it will become easy.

Start with Lateral Cervical Flexion to help you relax him and ease the horse into the *Head Up* position.

1. Begin with *Lateral Cervical Flexion.*
By now the horse should be comfortable with this. Standing on the left side, bring his nose toward you with your left hand, resting your right fingertips on his upper neck. Find the lateral position that is that the most comfortable for the horse, where his eyes will soften and his head drop just a little.

2. Rest the horse's head in the crook of your arm.
To get your left elbow under his jaw, keep your left *fingertips* on his nose, pivot your left elbow down in front of his nose and bring it up under and behind his chin. By keeping the fingers of your left hand on the opposite side of his nose as you do this, you can keep him from moving his head away. Gently rest your right hand on the top of his atlas. Keep your hands soft.

With the bars of his jaw resting in the crook of your elbow, gently lift his head. Do this little by little. Lift a little, relax a little. Feel your way through it. This will encourage him to let the weight of his head rest more and more on your arm (fig. 5.20). Watch his eyes as you do this.

Some horses will not have enough range of movement to allow them to relax their head comfortably on your shoulder. In this case, let them stay in the crook of your arm.

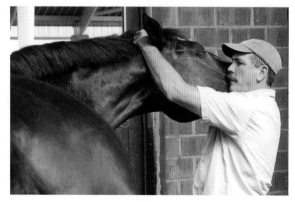

5.19 The goal is to take the weight of the horse's head on your arm or shoulder.

3. Rest the horse's head on your shoulder.

If the horse's head starts feeling heavy or if you are working on a tall horse, gently slide your shoulder under his chin while keeping the muscles relaxed. Keep your right hand on his poll or neck so that you can ask him to stay with you. Let the horse rest his head on your shoulder. Continue to watch the eye if your position allows. With any of these Techniques, you need to find the most comfortable position for the horse, wait ("feel") for him to relax there, then move forward with the Technique.

4. What to do once his head is up.

There are four things you can do once the horse's head is up. Which one (or ones) you use depends on the horse's comfort. Experiment and let the horse choose (fig. 5.21).

1. The first is, do nothing. Just supporting the weight of the horse's head alone for even a very short period of time will allow many horses to release huge amounts of tension in the poll and atlas. This can happen if you do nothing more than take the weight of the head for just a moment. Don't be in a hurry to start "doing" anything until the horse is as relaxed in this position as he can be. Give him a chance to relax before doing anything else.

2. The second is *Search, Response, Stay, Release.* This process works very well and is especially helpful in getting tense horses to relax in this position. By searching gently with your fingers around the poll and atlas and feeling and watching for responses, especially in the eye, he will let you know where to stay with your fingers and

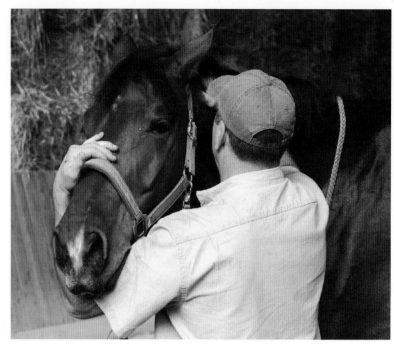

5.20 **Working with the horse's head in the crook of your arm.**

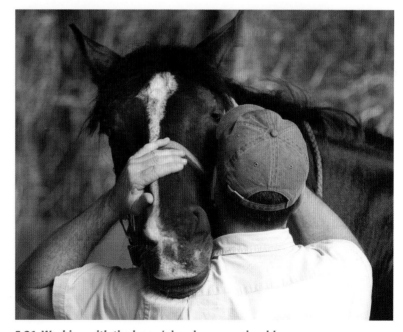

5.21 **Working with the horse's head on your shoulder.**

what pressure to use. He may ask for anything from an *air gap* to a *lemon* pressure massage (fig. 5.22). Take your time. Give him time to relax.

3. Thirdly, you can massage the muscles and tendons on top, around, and between the poll and atlas. Your pressure can range from *air gap* to

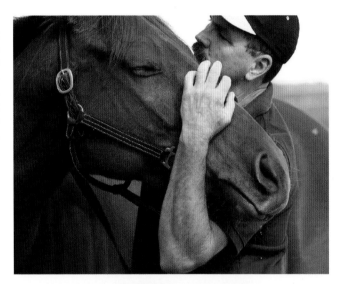

5.22 Using a very light touch to search for responses, find spots that will relax the horse even more.

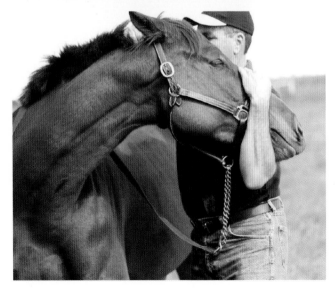

5.23 Once the horse is relaxed you can gently move the joints of the poll, atlas and upper neck through a gentle range of motion.

lemon—whatever he will allow—but if he begins to tense up, you are using too much. When you feel him relax more, you are on the right track and can go deeper. Feel for any knots or hardness in the muscles.

Real progress can be made once the horse is relaxed and endorphins kick in. You will notice his eyes softening or closing, possibly his nose twitching, his breath changing, and his head getting heavy as the muscles relax. Then you can massage these spots deeper.

4. Lastly, move the head *gently* through a range of motion. Use "The Principle of Release of Tension in a Joint or Junction" (p. 15).

When you move a joint or junction through its natural range of motion in a relaxed state, it releases tension in that junction. Once the horse is relaxed, slowly move the head and neck through a gentle range of motion (fig. 5.23). You can gently bend his poll and neck laterally by stepping sideways (you, not the horse). You may also flex the head and neck up and down by bending your knees, and then by standing up again. This will release tension in the poll, atlas, and rest of the vertebrae in the upper neck.

Do this slowly and feel for resistance in the movement. Remember, *resistance means restriction*. When you do feel resistance, soften your movement so that he can relax through the restriction. The horse has to be relaxed for this to be effective.

5. Step back and allow the horse to release.

Be aware that at some point the horse may need to step back so that he can release and really let the tension go. You can step back at any time then start again where you left off after giving the horse a small break. An example of when to do so could be after you have been doing this for anywhere from a minute to a few minutes with the horse relaxed, and suddenly he absolutely wants you to let his head go. In this case he probably needs a break so step back to allow him to "shake it loose."

Note: The horse can and will be releasing tension even as you are performing any of these Techniques. However, his nervous system may overload during a Technique and he will need a chance to process the release. When this happens he will usually let you know by persistently pulling away. This doesn't mean that you should step back every time he resists, *but you should be mindful of when he needs a break. Again, this is something you will get a better feel for as you practice on different horses.*

What Ifs?

■ *What if I am working on a tall horse?*

In this case you must ask the horse to come down to you. You do this by taking a small step backward after he has relaxed as much as he can on your shoulder, while keeping his head on your shoulder (fig. 5.24). Gently encourage him with your right hand behind his poll as you do this. He will have to extend his neck out and lower his head if he wants to continue to rest his head on your shoulder.

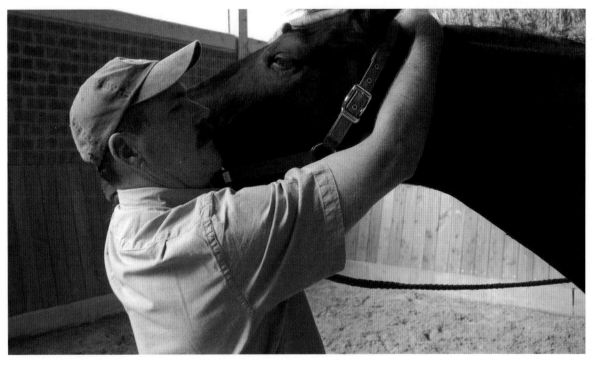

5.24 Take a small step backward to encourage a tall horse to lower his head to you.

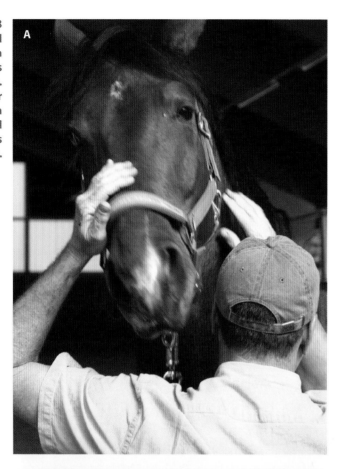

5.25 A & B Don't pull down when the horse raises his head (A). Keep your hand gently on his nose until he relaxes again (B).

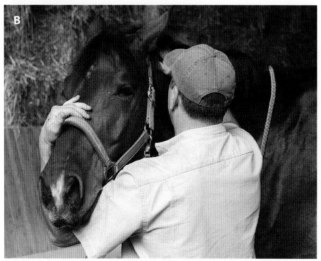

If you can take a small step backward and have him extend the neck out further it can have the added effect of softening the muscles behind the poll even more, but only if the horse is able to easily do this. Be aware that some horses will not yet be comfortable extending the neck out in this direction until they have loosened up in the poll, atlas, and throatlatch area.

■ *What if he pulls his head away?*

If the horse pulls back or tries to raise his head out of reach, resist the temptation to pull him down (figs. 5.25 A & B). You won't win that one.

Keep your hand gently on his nose and let him raise his head. You can't keep him from raising his head, but you can keep him from taking his head to the side by keeping your hand on his nose. Just keep his head "in the neighborhood" without pulling down on his nose until he realizes he's not going anywhere and brings his head back down.

■ *What if the horse won't relax onto my shoulder?*

Some horses relax easily into this position and others remain tense. Be patient. Take a deep breath, soften your hands, and wait. If the horse still isn't relaxing, try the following trick:

With the head still (somewhat) on the shoulder, search for a spot in the area behind the ear with the tip of one finger—*barely touching the horse's hair* (figs. 5.26 A–C). Search one hair at a time for a "blink." You may have to position your head so that you can see the eye from here. Once you get a blink, take a deep breath and stay very,

very lightly on that spot. *Resist the temptation to massage or push harder.* If you do, the horse will just block it out.

Keep your finger lightly on that spot. It may take a second, or it may take a minute, but if you stay light enough and long enough, the horse will start to relax onto your shoulder.

If you do this correctly (meaning *lighter-than-air gap* pressure), the horse will begin to let the weight of his head down on your shoulder, sometimes very suddenly.

Note: This may surprise you! But don't have a timetable on this one. If you stay light enough and long enough, the horse will have to let go.

■ ***What if the horse grinds his teeth or jaw while his head's on my shoulder?***

Often horses with a lot of tension in the neck and poll will grind their teeth as they relax this area. This is just a sign that something is happening. The horse will often do this while you are performing the *Lateral Cervical Flexion Technique* as well. The same as with fidgeting: When these happen, continue what you are doing. It is leading to a release. You will almost always find that they will only grind when they start to relax or "give in."

■ ***How long should I do this?***

As long as your horse stays relaxed, and you can continue to hold him up. However, always be mindful of the horse. Often he will relax to a certain point and then want to get out of the position or pull away. When this happens, he has

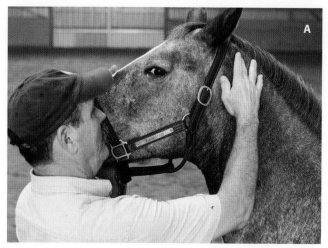

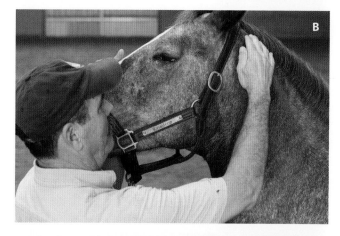

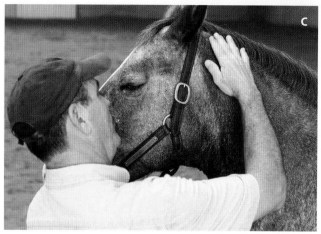

5.26 A–C Barely touch the area behind the ear with the tip of one finger, searching for a "blink" (A). Keep your finger there lightly (B), until the horse relaxes onto your shoulder (C).

relaxed down to where he can feel another level of tension. If you can persuade him to stay comfortably through it, okay, but if he really needs to be let go, step back and let him release. You can always start over where you left off.

- ■ *Why does my horse have pain or tension in the poll?*

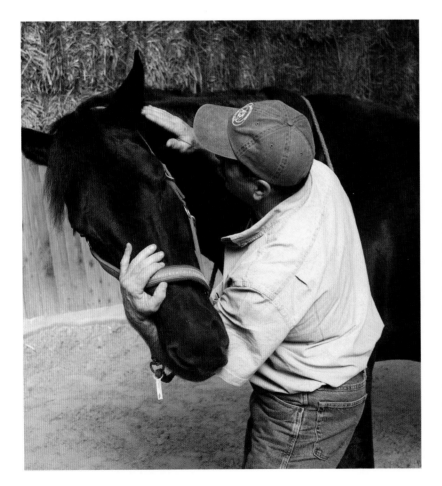

5.27 Step slightly to the side to relax the horse.

Over the years I have found correlations between pain issues in certain areas in the horse's body and pain or tension in the poll. These issues can range from the most direct, such as the horse hitting his head or pulling back while hard tied, to less obvious connections such as foot or lower leg pain corresponding to tension on one side of the poll or the other.

In my experience, there is a direct correlation between pain in the front feet and pain and tension in the poll and atlas. Pain from sore or even tender feet will radiate up through muscles that originate and insert between the head and foreleg such as the *brachiocephalic* and *omotransverse* muscles (see fig. 6.2, p. 64).

When the feet are sore, there is tension in the poll and atlas, especially if there is a chronic foot issue with soreness over an extended period of time. Frequently, after the problem or soreness in the feet has been taken care of, tension in the poll remains. This often shows up as head-shyness. So, when you release the tension in the poll, obvious changes in behavior, movement, and overall performance will result.

Horses with soreness in the front feet also have a tendency to be tense or restricted in the movement of other muscles of the neck and shoulders, the lower neck and Neck-Shoulder-Withers Junction (see p. 62). I will deal with this and the effects on the rest of the body in the next chapter.

I have also noticed a correlation between pain on top of the poll and pain in the back. Pain in the back can come from any number of things: from poor saddle fit, to compensating for pain in feet or legs, to injury. Compensating for discomfort in one part of the body creates tension patterns in other areas—and the back is one.

More often than you may think, pain, tension

and restriction in the *longissimus dorsi* muscle of the back results from riding habits that don't allow for proper movement in the back (see fig. 8.9, p. 152). When this muscle loses its ability to function—connecting the front and hind end of the horse in movement—muscles in other parts of the body that are compensating for this are affected.

Horses that are ridden "overflexed" in the poll over a long period of time will often be tight and overdeveloped in the area underneath the atlas, between the jaw and atlas. This usually goes along with extreme tightness in the sacral area, gluteals and hamstrings. As you can see, the whole horse is interconnected and this is why bodywork is so effective.

Tips

- As you bring the horse's head to the side in preparation for raising the head, feel for the lateral bend that is most comfortable for the horse. Some are more comfortable to the front, others more to the side. If he is on your arm or shoulder and you are having trouble getting him to relax, try stepping slightly to the side or more to the front as you search for a better position—for the horse, of course—(fig. 5.27).

- You may change the order of doing many of these Techniques. If you are having difficulty with any one of them, move to another, or do the same one on the opposite side. When you come back to the original Technique, the horse will often have released tension and it will be easier.

For example, a horse that is extremely head-shy often has difficulty relaxing when you start at the poll. In a case like this you can change the order of the Techniques and perform the next Technique, the *Scapula Release* (p. 62) to release tension in the Neck-Shoulder-Withers Junction first. This often relaxes the horse enough so you can work on the poll.

If you are having difficulty and keep trying to do the same Technique over and over again, the horse will quickly learn to evade what you are asking and just "go through the motions," not relaxed and not releasing tension.

As a rule of thumb, if you have tried three times to do a particular Technique without success, then move on to another one and come back to the original Technique afterward.

Note: *Have extra patience with horses that are head-shy. Ninety-nine percent of the time this is a sign of pain, discomfort, or tension. Even if you think it might only be a behavioral issue or memory of past traumas caused by hitting his head, ear-twitching (being controlled by twitching the ear rather than the upper lip), or pulling back on a halter, give the horse the benefit of the doubt.*

He cannot easily let go of pain or tension in the poll: He ends up blocking this pain rather than letting it go. Releasing this extremely important area of the horse can make the biggest difference in both performance and attitude. This is your opportunity to help him let go of pain and resistance in this area.

6

The Neck-Shoulders-Withers (C7-T1) Junction

Techniques 1 & 2:

- **SCAPULA RELEASE—** *DOWN AND BACK*

- **SCAPULA RELEASE—** *DOWN AND FORWARD*

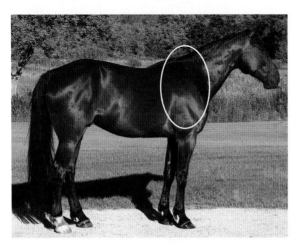

6.1 A & B Key Junction Number 2: The Cervical-Thoracic Junction.

Before You Begin

GOAL: To release and drop the scapula *down and back* and then *down and forward* in a relaxed state, beyond the normal relaxed range of motion.

RESULT: A release of tension in the muscles that attach the forelimbs to the body; deeper muscles of the junction of the neck and withers; and key muscles that affect both the poll and atlas, and the hind end. There is an improvement in range of motion in the front limbs; elasticity and "shock-absorption" function in the legs and shoulders; release of tension in the hind end; and more coordinated movement between the front and hind end.

WHERE YOU WORK—ANATOMY

Unlike humans, horses do not have a joint that connects the shoulder blade (scapula)—and thus the forelimb—to the body. The shoulder blade is attached to the horse's body by a complex system of muscles, fascia, and connective tissue, meaning there is no skeletal connection at all. You can picture this muscular system of attachment as a "sling" holding the trunk between the two forelimbs and providing support and movement. The neck joins the body at this junction also.

Major Skeletal Structures of This Junction

The horse's trunk consists of 18 (on some horses, 19) *thoracic verte-brae,* to which 18 corresponding ribs attach, forming the rib cage. The bottom ends of the most forward eight ribs are attached to the *sternum* (fig. 6.1 B).

The *scapula* is the shoulder blade of the horse. The *withers* are the *spinous processes* of the thoracic vertebrae from about T4 or 5 to T8 or 9, depending on the conformation of the horse (see fig. 6.40, p. 100). They are essentially long extensions of the vertebrae that "stick out" above the shoulder blades. Of course their function goes beyond "sticking out" and keeping your saddle—and you—from sliding off the horse: They are major anchoring points for muscles and ligaments that support the head and neck; act as a bridge that connects the front end to the hind end; and are part of the connection of the forelimbs to the body.

The *Neck-Trunk Junction (C7-T1 or Neck-Shoulders-Withers Junction)* is where the last vertebra of the neck joins with the first vertebra of the trunk. By releasing tension at this junction you release it in the whole area. *The Scapula Releases* are the first steps in dealing with tension in the muscles of this junction.

Major Muscles, Tendons, and Ligaments

The muscles, tendons, and ligaments of this junction are many. They also support the head, neck, shoulders, and trunk; move the forelimbs forward and back; brace before takeoff; help absorb impact when landing; and move and bend the head and neck, among other things. (The forelimbs bear the majority—60 to 65 percent—of the weight of the horse.)

They are strong, multilayered, and many lie under the scapula out of reach of your hands. Therefore, one of the best ways to release tension in this junction is to put the horse in a position that allows him to release it.

Equally important, from the point of view of the Masterson Method, are muscles that affect performance in other parts of the body. Two important front-end muscles that fall into this category are the *brachiocephalic* and the *omotransverse* muscles (fig. 6.2).

The *brachiocephalic* muscle originates at the base of the head near the atlas at the top end, and

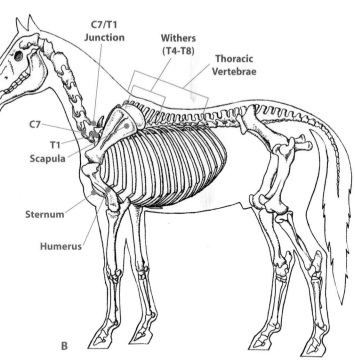

C7/T1 Junction · Withers (T4-T8) · Thoracic Vertebrae · C7 · T1 · Scapula · Sternum · Humerus · B

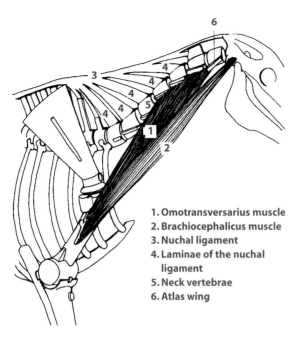

6.2 **Major parts of the neck.**

1. Omotransversarius muscle
2. Brachiocephalicus muscle
3. Nuchal ligament
4. Laminae of the nuchal ligament
5. Neck vertebrae
6. Atlas wing

inserts at the bottom end on the forearm (humerus, see fig. 6.1 B) below the shoulder. It has two basic functions: 1) When the head and neck are fixed it brings the foreleg forward, and 2) when the leg is fixed or anchored, it brings the neck downward and tilts the head up, as when the neck is extended.

The *omotransverse* muscle originates at the atlas and inserts at the humerus on the foreleg. It works with the brachiocephalic muscle to bring the leg forward and helps to raise the scapula. These two large muscles are also important in that they put tension on the poll and atlas and, as you know, when tension accumulates there it affects other parts of the body.

These muscles accumulate tension not only in the course of their normal job stated above, but also from pain in the feet and legs. (I discussed this earlier in "Why does my horse have pain or tension in the poll?" See p. 60.)

The last group of muscles that demonstrate the connection between this junction and other parts of the body are the *longissimus dorsi* muscles (fig. 6.3). These large, long muscles go down either side of the back and support, connect, and coordinate movement between the hind and front ends of the horse. They begin at the pelvis, run along the back on each side of the spine, and insert in the vertebrae of the lower neck just in front of the neck/withers junction. They are important locomotion muscles in all three (to five) gaits. Releasing restriction in these muscles has a direct impact on how the horse moves.

RELEASING TENSION: THE EFFECTS

Front-End Movement and Suspension

Range of motion of the forelimbs becomes restricted when muscles that are responsible for

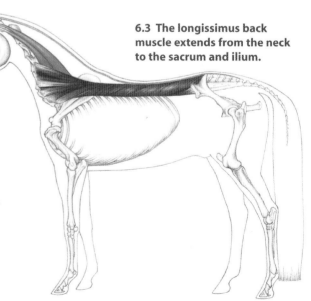

6.3 **The longissimus back muscle extends from the neck to the sacrum and ilium.**

moving the front leg forward and backward accumulate tension and are unable to release. Releasing this tension allows the horse to step out further and leads to a more fluid and extended gait.

In addition, when muscles that attach the forelimb to the body and support the front-end structure become tense, the horse loses his ability to absorb the impact of the foot hitting the ground and his ability to move with suspension. When this happens there is increased impact and load on the muscles, tendons, ligaments, and joints of the feet, legs, and shoulder. Thus, accumulation of tension in the *Neck-Shoulder-Withers Junction* can lead to issues in the feet and legs. Releasing tension here helps not only to improve range of motion but also prevents stress to joints, muscles and ligaments of the forelimbs.

Neck-Shoulder-Withers Junction and the Poll

I've already discussed the poll-front foot connection through the *brachiocephalic* and *omotransverse* muscles. When you release tension in the *Neck-Shoulder-Withers Junction,* you also release tension at the other end of these muscles—the poll and atlas—thus beginning the process of releasing tension in the rest of the body.

Neck-Shoulder-Withers Junction and the Hind End

When you release this *C7-T1 Junction* under the scapula, you are also affecting the hind end. I have described how the *longissimus dorsi* muscles attach to the pelvis at one end and in the lower neck under the scapula at the other end. In fact, you will often see the hind end relax or even kick when you release under the scapula (details later in this section). So you can see how releasing tension in this key junction affects how the horse's entire body works and moves together.

Now I will start to discuss the specifics of Technique 1: Scapula Release—*Down and Back.* Technique 2: *Down and Forward* starts in detail on page 80.

Case Study

This not only makes sense but is true. My partner and I had a client well known on the hunter-jumper circuit. He had a very good—and successful—jumper.

Some of these horses campaign hard and can get pretty sore, and this particular horse benefited from bodywork at least once each week. Veterinarians are regular visitors to show-jumping barns and stables to keep horses sound, especially in the feet and legs department. This horse was no exception.

How important this body-feet/leg connection is became apparent to me one day when my partner and I were chatting with one of the vets. He wondered out loud why he'd only been called once this season to deal with feet and leg issues with this horse, when the previous season he was treating something every couple of weeks. The answer was that by keeping the key junctions of the horse's body loose, his natural ability to absorb impact on the feet and legs was enhanced, thus reducing the need for veterinary treatment of the feet and legs.

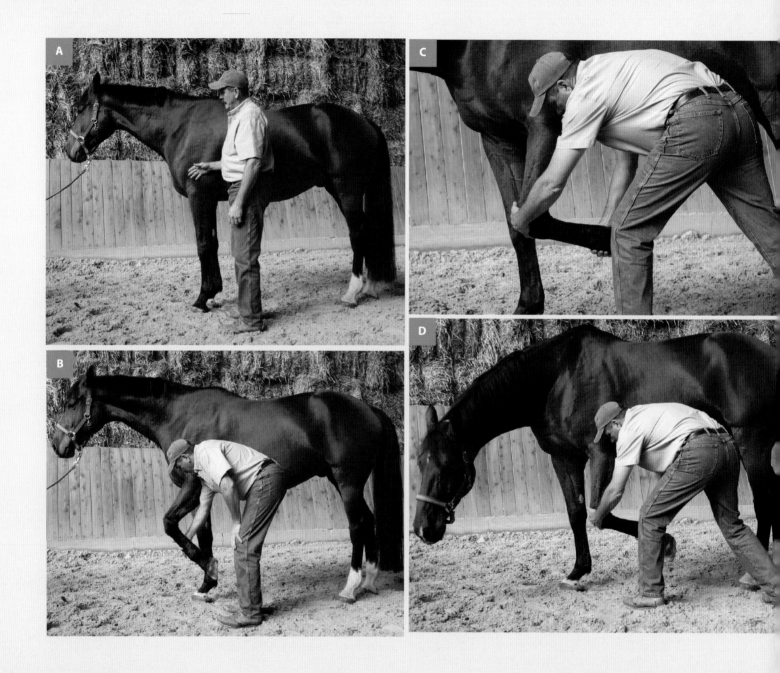

QUICK OVERVIEW: Step-by-Step

TECHNIQUE 1: SCAPULA RELEASE—*DOWN AND BACK*

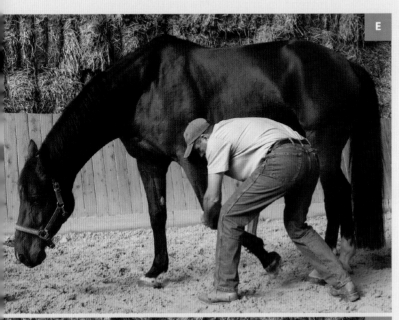

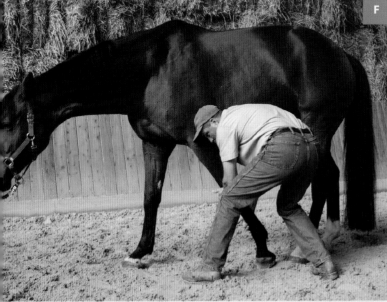

Step 1. Stand at the horse's shoulder, facing forward (A).

Step 2. Pick up the foot (B).

Step 3. Rest the horse's ankle in your right hand and place your left hand on the horse's knee (C).

Step 4. Allow the horse to relax the leg and shoulder as much as he is able (D).

Step 5. Slowly guide the leg down and back, straightening the leg and lowering the foot as you go (E). Don't forget to lower the foot!

Step 6. Encourage the horse to rest in this position as long as he can by keeping your hand on the leg or foot (F).

Technique 1 in More Detail

1. Position the horse.

Position the horse so that there is room for both of you to work. The best place is in the center, diagonally across the stall. As he steps back you don't want him to hit his rear end on the wall and bounce forward. In addition, when in the center, should he have a sudden urge to move, he has room to move away from you rather than *through* you.

It always helps to simply ask the horse to move *before* you begin working on him. Just by moving to where you want him he is *yielding to you* from the start. You're working together, both on the same page. Asking the horse to move his feet is a helpful trick when working with any horse.

Finally, make sure that the horse is standing somewhat square whenever you pick up any one of his legs. It's important he keeps his balance. You don't want him to have to step or fall into the position you're asking for before he is ready.

2. Position yourself.

With both *Scapula Releases* it's easier to bring a foot or leg toward you rather than push it away from you. So when you are asking the horse to release the leg down and *back,* you should be facing the *front* of the horse. When you are asking the horse to release the leg down and *forward,* you should be facing *back.* This allows you to bring the leg toward you in both cases.

So, with this first *Scapula Release—Down and Back,* stand at the horse's shoulder facing toward the front of the horse.

3. Support yourself.

It may help to rest your elbows on your knees to support your back while in this position.

You can also get down on one knee if you feel comfortable doing so next to the horse (fig. 6.5). This might make it easier on your back. However, make sure there is room for the horse to move away from you if he needs to move, and be prepared to move away from the horse if you need to.

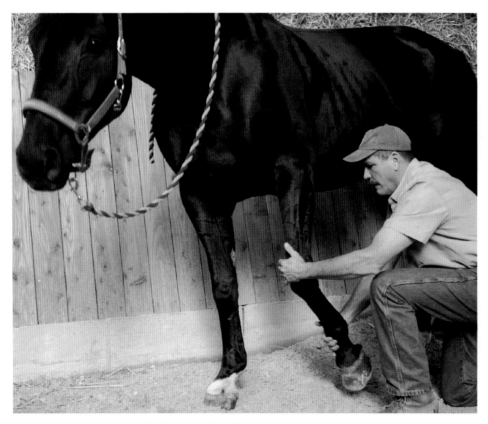

6.5 You can support your back by getting down on one knee.

4. Pick up the foot.

If facing forward and asking for the horse's foot is awkward, face the hind end and ask for the foot as if you were going to clean it, then turn and face forward while holding the foot.

On the left leg, facing forward, hold the leg with your right hand on the pastern and the knee with your left hand (figs. 6.6 A & B). On the right side, do the opposite. Hold the pastern in your left hand and the knee with your right.

Note: *It's important to place your hand on or above the ankle rather than below it. This leaves the foot dangling so it is easier for the horse to step down on it as you lower the foot. If you hold below the pastern, and keep the hoof up as you set the leg down, he may step on the pastern rather than the foot.*

Allow the horse to relax. This may take five seconds, or it may take 15. Support the weight of the leg. You can take advantage of this time to massage the flexor tendons, or do the "hoof rotation," that is, hold your hand flat across the bottom of the hoof or shoe, and move the hoof in a circular motion. This gently wiggles the leg, which relaxes the shoulder and the joints.

When you feel the horse has relaxed as much as he is going to, start guiding his foot down and back.

5. Pick a spot on the ground for the foot.

Use this point as a place to aim for, but also feel for what is comfortable for the horse as you lower the leg. You are looking for a little farther back than he would normally rest it on his own. The horse may easily be able to relax the foot down to this point, or he may not. You don't need to set

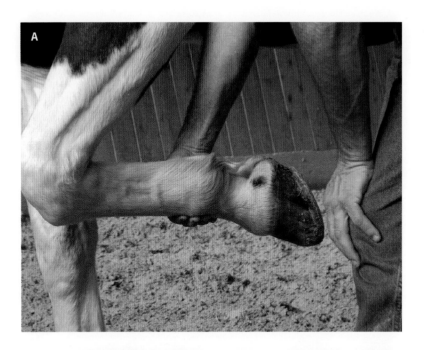

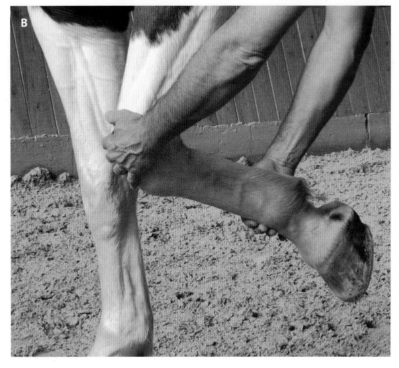

6.6 A & B Hold the pastern in your right hand, and the knee with your left.

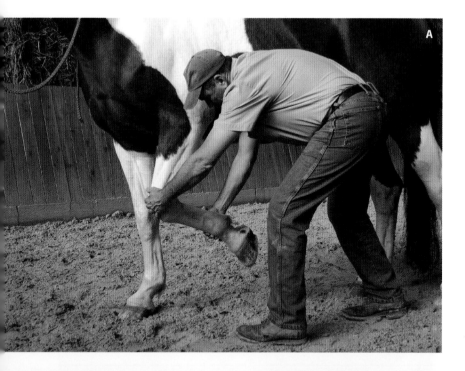

the leg back a long distance to get the release. If the spot you choose is too far for him to relax the leg comfortably into, he will keep picking it back up, When this happens, guide his foot down to a spot a little closer. (See the "What Ifs?" starting on p. 73.)

It's better to give him a more comfortable position that he can relax in longer than a more stretched position he has trouble relaxing into. Go where the horse is most comfortable. Some horses prefer going *straight back and under*, while others like, *back and out more to the side*.

6. Lower the leg down and back.

When you feel the horse has relaxed some of the weight of the leg in your hand, lower the hand that's holding the foot toward your spot on the ground.

Straighten his leg as you bring the foot down. Do this by using your "knee hand" to straighten his leg as you lower your "foot hand" toward the ground (figs. 6.7 A & B). Often the horse relaxes the leg as the knee straightens. Be sure to lower the foot toward the ground as you do this. Don't ask the horse to step back and set his foot down while holding his foot up. That just isn't fair!

This is not a stretch.

Remember that you are not pulling or stretching the leg back. You are supporting the leg until the horse relaxes it then guiding the leg down and back. The goal is to allow the scapula to drop just a little bit beyond where it would normally drop—*in a relaxed state.*

The scapula only has to drop an inch or so before the foot is down in order to release ten-

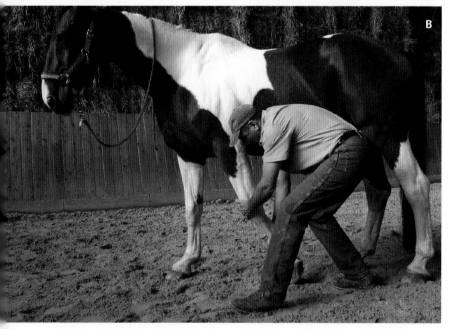

6.7 A & B Use your "foot hand" to aim his foot to a point on the ground (A). Use your "knee hand" to straighten the leg as he relaxes it down (B).

sion. Once you have a mental picture of where you want the foot to set down, get in the habit of looking at the "point of the shoulder" as you feel for the scapula to drop.

You will be able to see and feel when you get a slight drop. Remember, you only need to feel a slight relaxation for it to work.

7. Watch and feel for the release.

The release is visible. If you watch the point of the shoulder and the leg as you set the leg back, you can see the release movement. Also, when you know what to look for, you can see release responses such as eyes twitching, licking and chewing, and yawning.

The release is palpable. When your hands are on the leg you can feel when the horse lets go. When his foot is resting back on the ground, if there is not a lot of weight on it, you can gently wiggle the leg and shoulder to encourage the horse to relax it even more. If you wiggle the leg and he tenses, stop. If he has weight on the leg and you can't wiggle it, that's all right, too.

The longer he is able to relax in the foot-back position, the more he will release. Keep your hand on the foot or on the leg. Most horses will pick the foot back up when you take your hand off. You may slide your hand farther up the leg to give your back a break, but as long as your hand stays on the leg he will stay in this position longer.

Sometimes the horse will step back and hold his position, sometimes he will step back and then pick up the front leg, and sometimes he will step back and then step forward again. All of these are okay as long as you see or feel that he has relaxed and dropped the scapula before his foot reaches the ground. If you aren't sure this has happened, step back yourself for about 30 seconds and see what he has to say.

If your horse leaves the leg in this position then let him stay there until he steps out of it on his own. After stepping out of it, sometimes the horse will show you visible release responses right away, sometimes he will stand and process and then show releases after he is done. Sometimes he will show no responses at all. This depends on the horse, the amount of tension he may have had, how much he released, and whether he's comfortable showing it to you or not. The *Scapula Release* is a major endorphin releaser. Watch the horse's eyes after this release and you'll see what it means (fig. 6.8).

Release vs. Movement

There is a difference between an active movement of the scapula down and back when walking, for example, and when releasing the scapula:

- When the scapula drops down and back in normal active movement, the muscles involved in that movement are active.
- When you ask for the movement through a certain point in a relaxed state, the horse releases tension in the muscles involved.

This is also different from a passive stretch: In a passive stretch, you are doing the work. With these releases you are putting the horse in a position to "let go."

Case Study

I was once working on a horse in the stall who just didn't want to show any release responses in front of me. I knew he wanted to yawn, but as I would step back to see what he had to say after doing some work, he would clamp his jaw tight and look the other way. I could tell it was working because I could feel the releases under my hands.

Finally, after one Technique, he went over to his blanket that I had draped over the stall door. He stuck his head under it and yawned six or seven times in a row. This goes to show you how strong body language is in the herd!

The moral: Back up and give the horse some space.

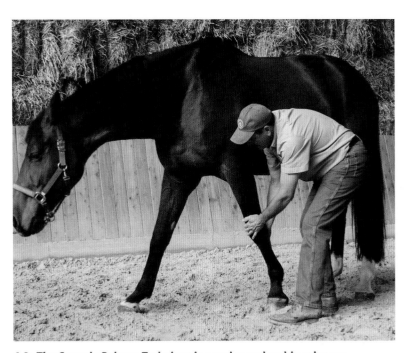

6.8 The *Scapula Release Technique* **is a major endorphin releaser.**

8. See what the horse has to say.

When you are finished take a step back to see what the horse has to say. You need to give him time to feel what has happened. Look for the release responses. You'll be surprised sometimes at the responses you get with the seemingly smallest drop of the scapula.

9. Give the horse space.

When you step back, step *way* back. The temptation is often to stand up close and pet the horse. However, some horses need more space than others to show you a release: They are more "self-conscious" while others just plain don't want to release in front of you. Release responses—licking and chewing for example—are signs of submission in the herd, and some horses don't want to show that.

Remember, as with all the Techniques, you are only looking for an improvement.

It is both safer and easier on the horse to do them gradually. This is your safeguard against injury—or aggravation of an existing injury. Don't have the mindset that a restriction is a problem and that you are going to "fix it." This causes resistance from the horse, which won't get you the release. By working in small increments and getting an improvement each time, you avoid the risk of hurting the horse.

Note: When processing the Scapula Releases, sometimes the horse will stay in the "release" position for anywhere from a few seconds to even a few minutes. This is not only because it feels good after having released tension but because his nervous system may be processing the release. It will appear that he is either staring off in the distance or he is half asleep. The difference is that his lips will twitch, his eyes will blink, or widen and then go to half-mast, and every once in a while his body will jerk as if he's received a little electric shock (fig. 6.9).

Stay calm! It is good to let the horse's nervous system process a bit. Synapses in the brain are re-firing as the nervous system lets the brain know that the restriction or soreness that it has been blocking out in that part of the body has released, and communication is reestablished between that part of the body and the brain.

Be patient and take your time. You'll be surprised how much improvement you can achieve in only a few sessions. You may notice when coming back to perform this exercise later that the leg feels easier to manipulate than when you first started out.

What Ifs?

■ *What if the horse refuses to let me lift the leg, or repeatedly pulls away?*

If the horse absolutely refuses, with his ears pinned back, there is probably a reason. It could be that he is guarding something in that leg, or there is discomfort or an injury in that leg, or in the opposite one, which is making it difficult for him to hold up the one you are working on. If that happens, move on to the next Techniques. You can always come back to this one later after you see how the horse behaves doing others.

If he still refuses and you suspect an injury, have a veterinarian look at the horse. It is a good idea to determine whether it is a stubbornness issue or not—that is, to make sure it isn't a veterinary issue.

■ *What if my horse won't relax the leg once I have it up?*

This is an indication that there is pain or restriction somewhere in the neck, shoulder, or withers, and the horse doesn't want to relax through it.

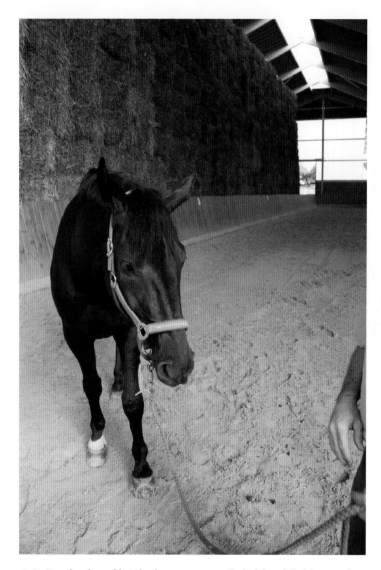

6.9 Step back and let the horse process. Twitching, blinking, and a "far-off" look in his eyes are signs of him processing a release.

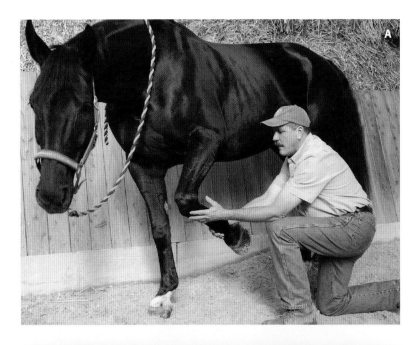

Supporting the weight of the leg more—even lifting slightly on the leg—may make it easier for him to relax it.

Don't be in a hurry. Be patient and wait for him to relax a little then slowly straighten the knee and guide it to the spot you've picked for that foot. The more time he can comfortably stay in the leg-back position, the better the release. However, it doesn't mean you've failed if he doesn't stay in this position.

If there is resistance to any move you ask of him, it is an indication that there is pain or restriction. This means that you need to help the horse release it. In general, when you run into resistance, soften slightly to give the horse a chance to relax the resistance slightly then move forward with the movement. In the case of the *Scapula Release,* to "soften" means you not only don't pull the leg, but you even lift it slightly to give the horse a chance to relax it before you move on. He may also resist if he feels your intention is to release the leg too far back. It will make it easier for him if the spot you have picked is a shorter distance rather than farther back (see next question).

■ *What if my horse begins to relax the leg down, then pulls it up?*

At some point while lowering the leg, the horse will likely pull the leg up. This is normal.

When this happens don't pull back on the leg. Keep your hands on the knee and ankle and go up with the leg a little thus "keeping him in the neighborhood" until he relaxes into your hand again (figs. 6.10 A & B).

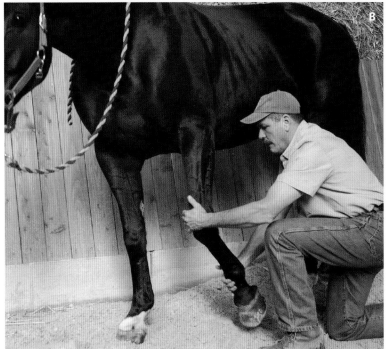

6.10 A & B When the horse "pulls up" go with him (A). Then, as he relaxes the leg, guide it down (B).

When the horse resists or starts to pull and you yield to it, he will usually stop pulling: You take away the resistance so the horse usually stops fighting it. Then you can continue and as he relaxes into your hand, be ready to guide the leg down to your "landing spot."

When he resists he has relaxed into a point of discomfort or restriction in the withers, scapula, sternum, or somewhere in this junction that he normally moves through in a non-relaxed state. This discomfort causes him to resist and pull the leg up.

Another thing that happens is that each time he pulls his leg up, he is releasing some ten-

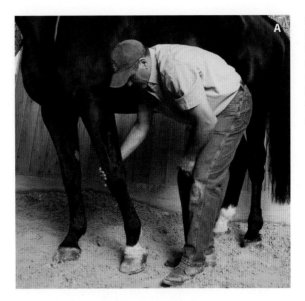

6.11 A & B
Release the leg to a spot that's not too far back (A). Set the foot back a little farther the second time (B).

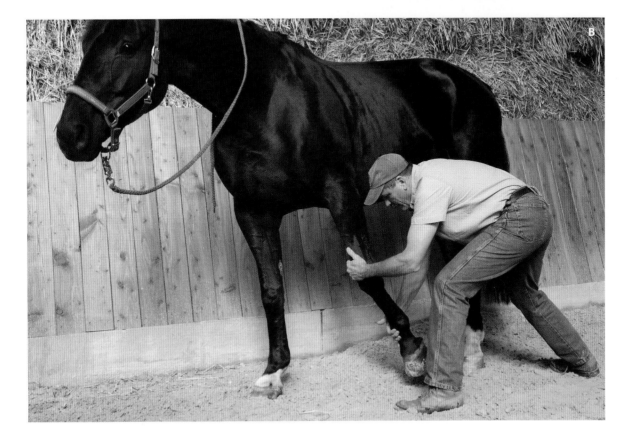

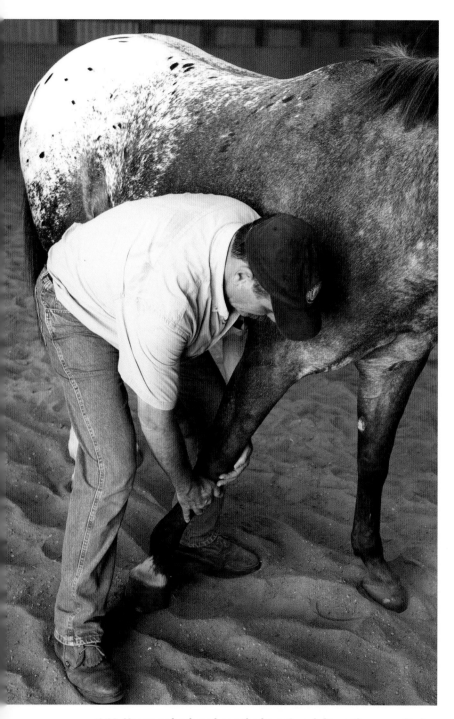

6.12 Use your body to keep the horse's weight on the opposite leg.

sion or restriction. This may happen a few times in a row, depending on how much tension or restriction is there. Each time you will feel the leg more relaxed.

If he continues to pull the leg up, or you feel that he is not relaxing the leg each time, you may be asking him to step too far back. In this case pick a spot for him that is a *shorter* distance back. Once he has released the leg down into this easier position, you can ask him to release the leg back farther a second time (figs. 6.11 A & B).

Note: Yielding to Resistance. Try this at home! Stand facing a friend. With one hand, hold on to her wrist. Pull gently on her arm and ask her to pull back. The second you feel her pull, push toward her and she will stop pulling. This is what happens with the horse if you yield quickly enough, and it may save you a lot of grief when asking the horse to move through a point of discomfort.

Caveat! It's important when yielding to resistance in the horse that you not take your hand off the horse whenever he pulls away or resists. If you do, the horse will learn (instantly) to do the same thing over again. HE will be training YOU to take your hands off and stop doing what you were doing!

■ *What if my horse quickly steps back and puts all of his weight on the leg without relaxing it?*

Sometimes the horse just thinks that's what you're asking him to do. Slow the process down, as if you were asking him to gently set the foot down. If you can keep his weight on the opposite leg just a little longer as he puts this one down, it will give him a little bit more of a chance to release the leg as he does this. Each time it will get easier for the horse. All you are looking for at each step of the way is an *improvement:* Don't try to get it all in one go.

Be sure that the horse is standing square when you pick up the leg and that you're not asking him to step too far back or pulling him off balance. When you ask the horse to position any leg you have to allow him to keep his balance on the other three legs.

If he is setting it down right away because it is uncomfortable for him to relax it down, you can use your body weight to encourage him to keep his weight on the opposite leg just an instant longer (fig. 6.12). Stand in close to him when you ask for the leg. You don't need to pick up the foot, just shift his weight to the opposite leg and slide the foot back. Use your shoulder to hold him on the opposite leg long enough for him to release the scapula down. This creates a short delay that allows (fools) him into dropping the leg before he steps down on it. This will help him to release it.

■ *What if my horse does not want to rest the leg in this position once the foot is down? Does this mean he did not release?*

One reason he may not stay in this position is that there may still be tension here and he is unable to relax comfortably. There may still be layers of the onion to peel. In this case, ask again, and use your weight to keep his weight on the other leg just a little longer.

Remember, you don't have to make the restriction release all at once. You can "peel the onion" layer by layer.

Another reason is that he may not be entirely comfortable with a human in his stall doing these strange things with his legs. All horses are different. One horse may readily accept someone coming into his stall, messing with his legs and finding all of his sore spots. Another may be more defensive and guarded and will not want to *show* the release responses or processing in front of anyone after you have got the release.

However, if you do the Techniques with the horse in as relaxed a state as he can be, then he *will* release some tension, even if he doesn't show it to you.

A lot of these things will become more apparent to you after you have done this a few times, so don't be discouraged. If you are doing these Techniques even close to the descriptions in this book, the horse will release.

■ *How many times should I repeat this exercise within one session?*

If the horse can easily do what you're asking and relaxes his leg down in one try, once is enough.

If the horse has difficulty with it, you may want to do this a few times, feeling for an improvement each time. In this case, try to go slower the second time, giving the horse a chance to relax into the release.

■ *What if the horse has trouble relaxing?*

As with the previous question, often one session isn't enough. Every horse is different; has different issues, levels of tension, body type, etc. Some horses hold on to tension more than others. You may notice this reflected in their personalities. As

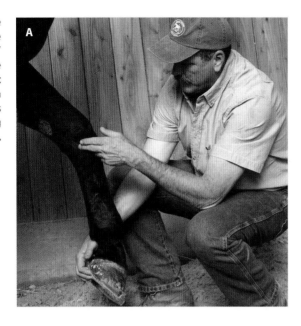

6.13 A & B The location of the "magic button," inside the knee (A). Tap the magic button when the horse has trouble releasing the leg (B).

long as you make an improvement each time, you are making progress.

Tips

- You don't have to do this leg release all at once. This is the case with most of these Techniques. Get a smaller release, then another. You will notice that each time you do this the movement will be more relaxed, and each time it will be easier for him to do the exercise. You're peeling layers off of the onion.

- It also helps to break it up a little by going from one side to the other, or doing another

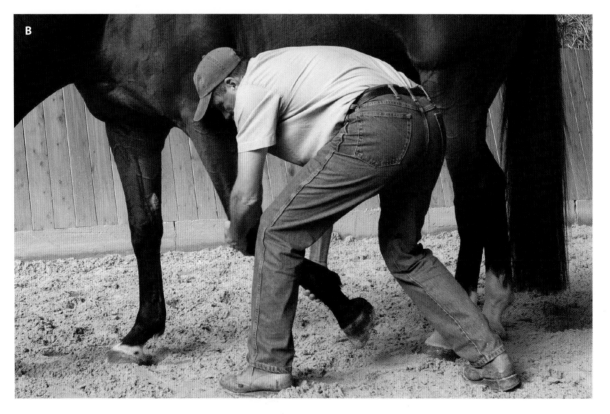

Technique and then coming back to this one. Don't become obsessed with doing it over and over to get it right. When you repeat the same thing more than two or three times in a row, the horse quickly learns to either go through the exercise without relaxing through it, or simply to evade the exercise.

In most cases you won't release *all* of the tension in one session, especially when the horse is in work, or whatever is causing the tension is still there. But you will make an improvement each time. Each time you repeat a Technique, or a session with the horse, look (or feel) for the improvement.

■ One more trick. There is a "magic button" inside the knee of some horses that you can tap (figs. 6.13 A & B). It is just below the bony protrusion on the inside of the knee. If you were to bend the knee, it would be in the hinge where it bends.

When the horse can't quite let the leg go, gently tap this spot with the fingertips of your "knee hand," which should already be in position on the knee. Tapping this point triggers a reflex response in the horse to "let go."

On the next page, I start Technique 2: Scapula Release—*Down and Forward*.

What to Do After a Bodywork Session

After working on a horse it's best to let him move freely for a while to "reset" his muscle memory and regain his coordination. Turnout is ideal. The horse naturally moves the muscles and junctions that he needs to in the way that he needs to. He may even roll around a bit and do his own "adjustments." Hand-walking is another alternative when turnout is not an option. If you prefer to ride, an easy ride on a loose rein works best.

As a general rule, it is best not to ask the horse's muscles to do whatever created the unwanted tension patterns to begin with before they've had a chance to experience a short vacation. How long a vacation depends on how much work was done on the horse. If you've only done a little, an afternoon off will do. If you've done a lot, and the horse had a lot of tension to release, a day off—or even two days—would be better. However there are horses on a training schedule that need to be ridden: In these cases, ride as lightly as possible. Many of the horses I work on that regularly show or compete are ridden or even shown the same day as the workout. Then again, these horses often get bodywork on a regular basis.

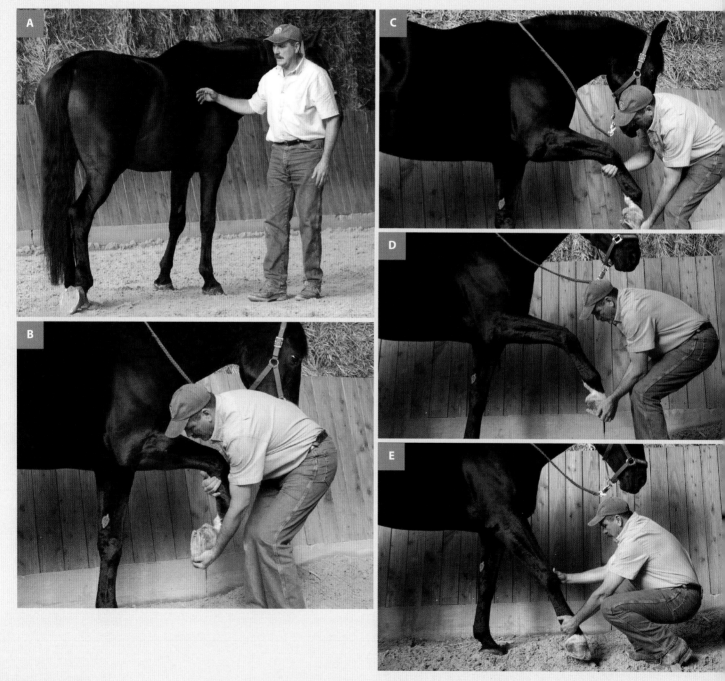

QUICK OVERVIEW: Step-by-Step

TECHNIQUE 2: SCAPULA RELEASE—*DOWN AND FORWARD*

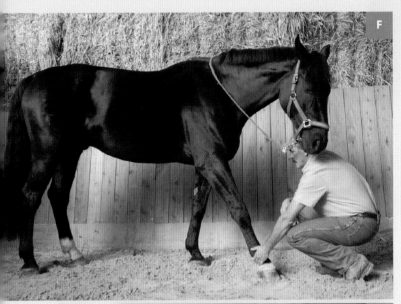

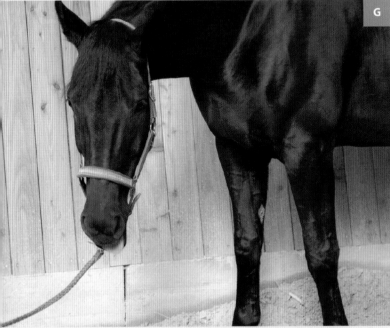

Step 1. Stand in front of the horse's shoulder, facing the hind end (A).

Step 2. Pick up the foot, bringing the leg forward (B).

Step 3. Take a small step backward and support the leg, holding the leg either by the toe or with your hand under the pastern (C).

Step 4. Support your weight on your knees to protect your back, if needed, as you allow the horse to relax the leg. Pick your landing spot while you wait (D).

Step 5. Shift your hand to under the pastern and set the foot down in a line straight from the horse's knee (E).

Step 6. Keep your hand on the horse's foot to encourage him to relax in this position, if he will (F).

Step 7. Step back and see what the horse has to say (G).

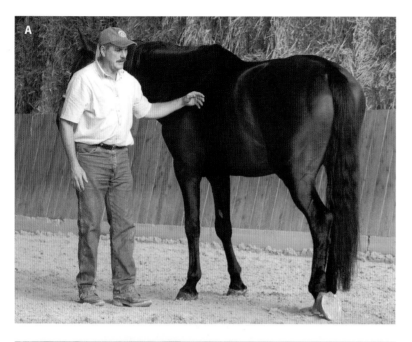

Technique 2 in More Detail

1. Position the horse.

Position the horse so that there is room for both of you to work. You want to make sure that you have room to bring the leg forward. Again, the best place is diagonally across the stall, but this time with his rump a little farther back toward the corner. And again, in the center of the stall, the horse has room to move *away* from you if he feels the need to move.

It always helps to ask the horse to move his feet before you begin working with him. When you move the horse to the position you want, he is yielding to you from the start. You're now both on the same page.

Make sure that the horse is standing reasonably square when you pick up his leg. When you ask him to release the leg down and forward, you *don't* want him to *fall* forward.

2. Position yourself.

Position yourself so that it will be easy for you to bring the leg forward. When picking up the leg to release forward, stand to the side, and *in front* of the horse's shoulder, facing *back*.

3. Bring the leg forward.

When you pick up the foot it will be easier to bring it *forward* if you are already standing forward of the shoulder. Ask the horse to pick up the foot as if you were going to clean the hoof. As soon as he lifts his foot, put one hand under the knee and bring the leg forward. You will have to take a step or two backward to bring his leg out in front (figs. 6.16 A & B). As you step

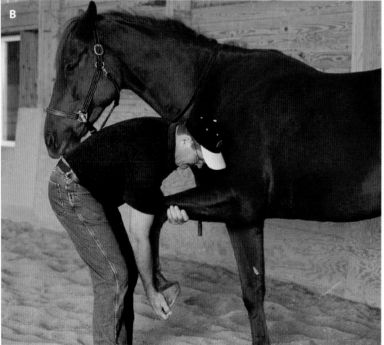

6.16 A & B Stand a little in front of the shoulder when you pick the leg up (A). Step backward and bring the leg forward (B).

back, you will need to be ready to support the weight of the leg.

4. Support the weight of the leg.
The best and safest way to do this is to get used to holding the foot by the toe (fig. 6.17). There are some good reasons for this:

a) The toe gives you the best grip, so it's easier for you to support the weight of the leg.

b) Since you have a firm grip on the toe, it's easier for the horse to relax into your hand.

c) The horse has a natural tendency to flex or pull back on the leg when you are not holding him below the ankle or pastern. When you have the toe, it's more difficult for the horse to pull back. Once his ankle "breaks over" he has the leverage to pull away. If you can keep him from doing this, it's easier for him to relax into your hand (fig. 6.18).

5. Support yourself.
Once you have the leg supported under the toe, rest your elbows on your knees to support your back (see fig. 6.17). The horse may be able to rest comfortably in this position, or he may not. Some horses fall forward and put their weight into your hand. Others hold the leg in that position with little support. By having the toe and your back braced you will be able to support the leg in either case.

6. Allow the horse to relax.
Hold the leg up long enough for him to relax in this position. This may be five seconds, or 25 seconds.

When you feel he has relaxed then you are ready to lower the foot to the ground.

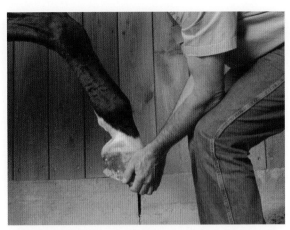

6.17 Holding the foot by the toe gives the horse support and you, leverage.

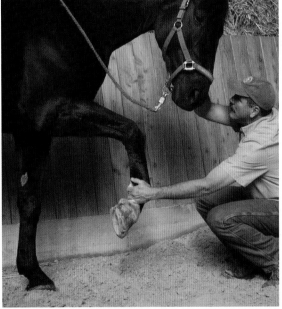

6.18 Not only does grabbing the horse by the ankle or foreleg give him no support, it also provides *him* leverage to pull away.

7. Pick a spot on the ground for the foot.
Pick a point on the ground to place the foot. It's important not to extend the leg too far forward. As a rule of thumb place the foot down at a point in a line straight down from the horse's knee.

If you keep bringing the foot forward as the horse lets the leg out, the horse will either: a) pull

6.19 Do not let the horse fall forward or hyperextend.

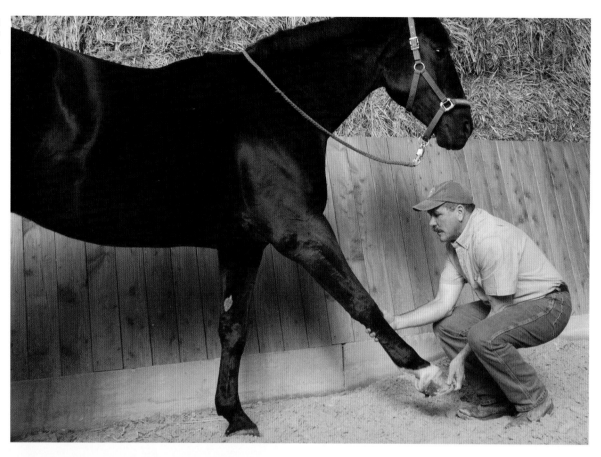

6.20 A & B Lift under the fetlock and remove your fingers from under the toe before setting the foot down (A). You can slip your hand under the heel as you set the foot down (B).

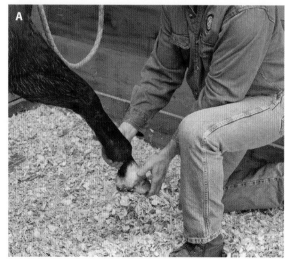

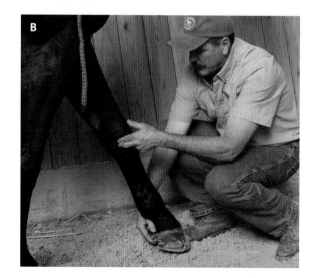

his leg back when he realizes it is too far, thus ending the *relaxed-state* part of the Technique, or, b) fall forward.

Note: Its important not to let the horse fall forward. There is a tendency when first doing the Scapula Release—Down and Forward to continue bringing the foot out and away from the horse until he either falls forward or has to pull back. If he falls forward and you can't support his weight, you must set the foot down before he hyperextends. Beware of this and set the foot down if you find him coming off balance (fig. 6.19).

8. Continue to support the weight of the leg as you lower it to the ground.
This is not a stretch: You are not pulling or stretching the leg out but supporting the leg until the horse relaxes, then guiding the leg down. The goal is to allow the scapula to drop just a little bit beyond where it would normally drop—*in a relaxed state.*

9. Shift your hand from under the toe to behind the ankle, or under the fetlock.
When you are ready to set the foot down, continue to support the toe with one hand while slipping the other hand under the fetlock. Lift slightly to support the leg by the fetlock before taking your fingers out from under the toe (figs. 6.20 A & B).

10. Go where the horse is most comfortable.
Feel for what is comfortable for the horse as you lower the leg in order to keep him relaxed. If he has trouble reaching the spot you have chosen, guide his foot down to a point a little closer in.

Some horses will be more comfortable going straight forward, others a little out to the side.

11. Watch, feel, and look for the release.
As with relaxing the leg back, the scapula only has to drop an inch or so before the foot is down in order to release tension. Get in the habit of looking at the point of the shoulder as you feel for the scapula to drop (fig. 6.21). You will be able to see and feel when you get a slight drop. Remember you only need to feel a slight relaxation as the foot comes down to get a release. Once the foot is resting on the ground, keep your hand on the

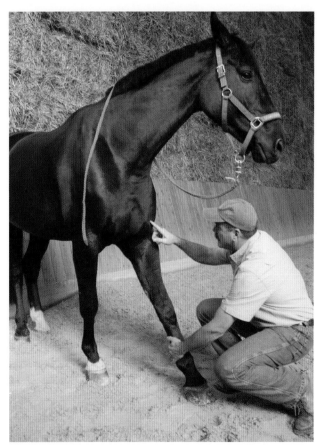

6.21 Look for the point of the shoulder to drop.

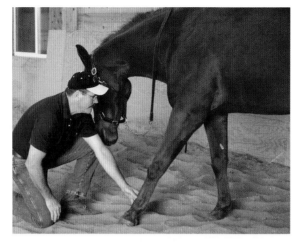

6.22 Keep your hand on the foot or on the leg to encourage the horse to stay in this position.

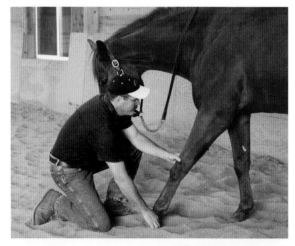

6.23 You can gently wiggle the leg if the horse stays relaxed.

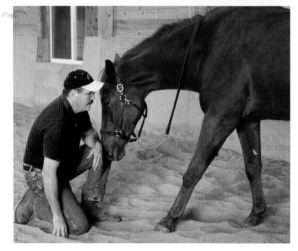

6.24 Allow the horse to stay in this position as long as he wants.

foot or on the leg to encourage the horse to stay in this position (fig. 6.22). Most horses will pick the foot back up when you take your hand off the foot or leg.

11. Gently wiggle the leg.

If there is not a lot of weight on the leg you can gently wiggle it and the shoulder to encourage the horse to relax even more (fig. 6.23).

If you wiggle the leg and he tenses, stop. If he has weight on the leg and you can't wiggle it, let him relax in that position.

The goal is to have the horse *remain standing with his weight on the opposite foot while relaxing this one on the ground.* The longer he is able to relax in this position the more he will release. So it's important to give him a comfortable position that he can relax in longer, rather than a more stretched position that he has trouble relaxing into.

If the horse leaves the leg in this position, let him process through the release until he steps out of it on his own (fig. 6.24).

12. Take a step back to see what the horse has to say.

Allow at least 20 or 30 seconds for him to "feel" what is going on the first time (fig. 6.25). Give him some space: Some horses need more than others to really relax. Watch his eyes for the signs of "processing" the release. The *Scapula Release— Down and Forward* will be a hard one for him to ignore.

Note: *These Scapula Releases can be done in a kneeling position next to your horse—if you are comfortable doing this; it may be a little easier on* your back (fig. 6.26). However, be aware that if the horse needs to move suddenly he will need space so you must be able to move out of his way.

Tips

- The same "magic button" mentioned under the Tips for *Technique 1: Scapula Release—Down and Back* (p. 66) on the inside of the knee can be used to help the horse release the leg down and *forward*. Just as the horse is ready to set the foot down, there may be resistance sometimes. Gently tapping this spot will trigger a reflex release that helps the horse to relax the leg that last little bit (see figs 6.13 A & B, p. 78).

- Break it up: Don't do the same thing more than two or three times in a row or the horse will catch on to what you are asking and just start going through the moves. Break up the sequence by going from one side to the other, or going back to a little light *Lateral Cervical Flexion* in between.

- Again, you don't need to set the leg forward a long distance to get the release. If it's too uncomfortable for the horse, pick a spot that is a little closer. The longer he can stay comfortably in this position, the more he will release. You can ask him to set the foot back a little farther a second time.

- And remember, you are only looking for *an improvement* each time you do this.

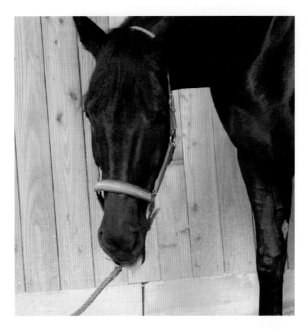

6.25 This Technique can also be a very powerful endorphin releaser for the horse.

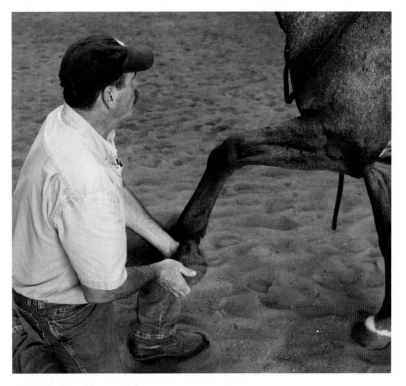

6.26 The kneeling position.

What Ifs?

Many of the questions about *Scapula Release—Down and Forward* have been answered in the *What Ifs?* section under *Scapula Release—Down and Back* (p. 73). However, there are differences in the way some of these issues are handled when bringing the leg *forward*:

■ **What if my horse begins to relax the leg down then pulls up?**

As with the previous Technique, at some point this will happen. As you are asking the horse to relax the leg down, in most cases, he will pull up before his foot reaches the ground. This is the point of restriction that you are helping the horse to move through. But you have to help him do it in a relaxed state (for him, not you!). The best way to do this is to hold the foot by the toe so that you can,

a) Yield and go up with the leg without losing control of the leg.

b) Be in a position to support his weight when he stops pulling and he relaxes into your hand.

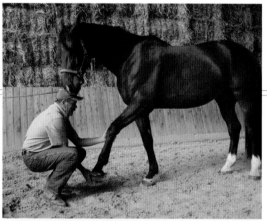

Holding the Horse's Foot by the Toe

Handling the foot by the toe is the best way to do this work with most horses. However, it's important to keep in the back of your mind when to let go. Always keep the foot well away from the ground and keep in the back of your mind an "invisible floor" below, where you will let go of the toe. This could be about a foot off the ground. If the horse leans into your hand and you drop your hand lower than this invisible floor, release the fingers that are holding the toe and let the leg down with the other hand (figs. 6.27 A & B).

6. 27 A & B Shift from under the toe to under the pastern as you lower the foot.

When you feel the horse begin to even slightly pull back or lift up on the leg, support the leg up toward the shoulder giving him the opportunity to relax the shoulder. Once you have all the weight, you can start to lower it again. This will allow him to relax through that point of restriction and be able to more comfortably drop the scapula. This may happen a couple of times before he is able to relax the leg down completely.

When you feel or anticipate tensing, support the leg up toward the shoulder to relax the leg *then* continue down. You may have to do this a couple of times on the way down. If the leg gets heavier, or your back gets sorer, you can put the leg down, rest, and start again where you left off. Any of these Techniques can be done successfully in increments.

As mentioned earlier, it may also make it easier for the horse if you only ask him to set the foot down a short distance forward rather than a longer distance. Remember to pick a starting point straight down from the knee.

■ *What if my horse quickly steps forward and puts all of his weight on the leg without relaxing it?*

First, be sure that the horse is standing square when you first pick up the leg, and that you're not asking him to step too far, or are pulling him off balance. When you pick up any leg you have to allow the horse's other three legs to keep his balance.

Second, you can to some degree preempt his falling forward by having a solid grip of the toe, stepping in closer into the horse, and pushing up on the leg to keep the horse's weight on the other

three legs (fig. 6.28). Be ready to do this if it happens more than once, or if you suspect it *might* happen.

Do not continue to bring the foot out and let the horse hyper-extend. If the horse is just too heavy, immediately set the foot down and start over again, this time asking for only a short distance forward.

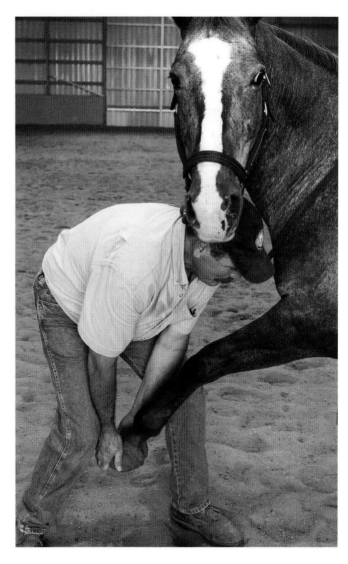

6.28 Push upward on the leg to keep the horse from falling forward and hyperextending.

Note: As with the Leg Back, you can use your body to keep him on the opposite leg just a bit longer, giving him the chance to release the shoulder before putting all of his weight on it. It is a little different in this Leg Forward position.

When releasing the left side, stand in close to the horse facing back, with the point of your left shoulder against the point of the horse's left shoulder. Place your left leg in front of, and across, the midline of the horse (fig. 6.29). Lean your shoulder against the horse's shoulder and gently ask him to shift his weight over as you encourage him to pick up the leg. You don't need to actually pick up the foot, but can slide his leg forward about a foot as you use your shoulder to keep his weight on the opposite leg for just a second. This will give him a chance to relax the shoulder down in a way that is much more comfortable, especially if there is a lot of tension or discomfort in this junction that he is trying to protect.

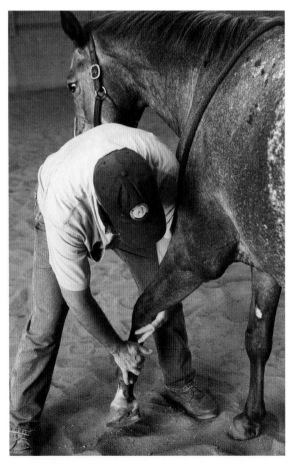

6.29 Use your shoulder to keep the horse's weight on the opposite leg.

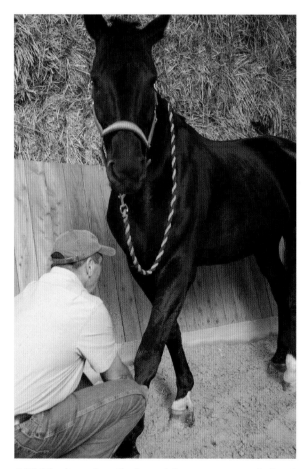

6.30 It's okay when the horse's leg crosses over in front.

■ *What if my horse paws or keeps pulling the foot out of my hand?*

Again, having the foot by the toe is the best way to start. The next step is to yield to the resistance the moment you start to feel it. Practice yielding to resistance with your friend again (see p. 00 [earlier]). It is a little more difficult, however, with pawing. Once a horse starts pawing, it can be a little more difficult to get him to stop as it works so well for him. If it becomes dangerous, it may become necessary to discipline the horse or train him not to paw, or to move on to another Technique. If the pawing is to protect a discomfort issue, then sometimes moving on through the session will relieve some of this.

■ *What if his foot crosses over in front?*

Guide the foot down wherever is most comfortable for the horse. Due to conformational factors or muscle-tightness issues, different horses are comfortable resting their feet in different positions. The best place to start with any Technique is where the horse is most comfortable, then to help the horse gradually move out from there in a relaxed state. Crossing over the midline in front is good for the horse (fig. 6.30).

■ *Can I ask the leg to come out to the side?*

Yes. If the leg is relaxed, you can slide the toe out

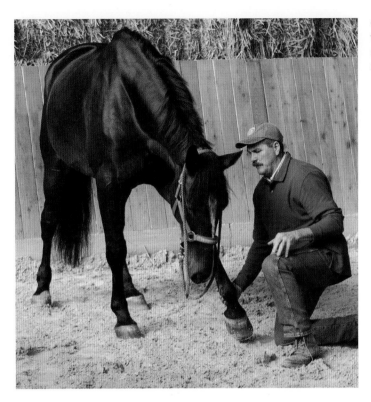

6.31 You can slide the toe out to the side to release tension laterally.

to the side (laterally) to release tension in this position. It's important that you not pull or force the leg out, especially if the horse pulls back. But when he is relaxed you can release tension in the *sternum, pectorals and other muscles of the shoulder* by relaxing the leg back, out to the side, and across the front (fig. 6.31). Just remember not to force the issue. Horses have to relax into these positions.

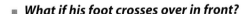

Note: *Be aware of possible discomfort or injury farther up in the neck, shoulder and withers, or in the opposite leg that may make it difficult for the horse to hold the leg up, or in the position you want. If there is doubt it's always best to err on the side of caution.*

Technique 3:
UNDER THE SCAPULA—C7-TI JUNCTION RELEASE

Before You Begin

GOAL: To access under the scapula for movement where the last vertebra of the neck joins the body—the *Cervical-Thoracic Junction*—and to release tension in major muscles of the junction.

RESULT: A release of tension in deeper muscles that affect movement of both forelimbs, neck, back, and hind end by asking for movement in this junction. This further improves the shock-absorber ability of the front end, the release of tension in the poll, and cooperation between the front and hind ends.

WHERE YOU WORK—ANATOMY

You first released tension in the vertebrae of the neck with the *Lateral Cervical Flexion Technique* (p. 33). Then with the three *Scapula Releases* described in this chapter, you use the limbs to ask the horse to release tension in the large muscles that attach the limbs to the

body. This *Neck-Withers Junction Release* is in a sense a continuation of *Lateral Cervical Flexion*, but now that you have released tension in the scapula you can work under it in the area of the last vertebra of the neck.

C7 is the lowest vertebra of the neck. T1 is the first vertebra of the trunk. *The C7-T1 Junction* is where they join. As you saw in the last chapter, the withers are part of the trunk vertebrae from T4 through T8. The thoracic vertebrae from T1 to T3 are "hidden withers," buried within muscles underneath the scapula of the horse.

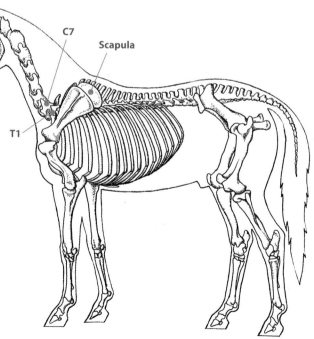

6.32 The Cervical-Thoracic (C7-T1) Junction.

The lower ends of these thoracic vertebrae—T1 to T8—join the sternum. This whole structure forms the main part of the trunk (thorax) of the horse.

All of the muscles that you have been working on with the *Scapula Releases* as well as the neck and poll muscles are affected by this Technique. These include the *longissimus dorsi, brachiocephalic, omotransverse, omohyoid* and *sternomandibular* muscles (see pp. 63 and 64). Major muscles involved in movement and stabilization of the forelimbs and withers "let go" with this Technique, and a further release of important muscles associated with the sternum such as *pectorals* and *deep pectorals* is achieved.

In short, you are going deeper into this junction with this Technique.

RELEASING TENSION: THE EFFECTS

There is also a neurological effect that releasing this junction has on the body. You will have noticed the "processing" that often takes place after the *Scapula Releases*. Asking for movement in the *C7-T1 Junction* after releasing the scapula, neck, and poll creates an even more profound release and often helps with longstanding front-end problems.

As you've seen, the *longissimus dorsi* muscles also insert in this area. This Technique further releases tension in the hind end.

Technique 3 in More Detail

You have already taken the first steps to releasing the *C7-T1 Junction* by having done the *Poll, Neck,* and *Scapula Releases*. One of the palpable indica-

tors of a successful Technique here is the relaxing of the *brachiocephalic* muscle where it crosses over this junction. This is one reason it helps to release as much of the other end of this muscle (at the poll) as possible before taking on this release.

So the first advice for this Technique is to do the other *front end releases*.

The second thing to know is that you may be using a little more force and pressure than you do for previous Techniques. This is where all of the sensitivity, strength, and skill that you have developed with Techniques thus far will come into play.

1. Position the horse.
Make sure there is room for both of you to work. Again, the best place is diagonally across the stall. You will be asking the horse to flex his neck toward you, but you may also ask the horse to take a step or two laterally so it's best not to place the horse against or near the wall.

Again, if you have a horse that is a little stubborn, reluctant, or nervous, it helps to ask the horse to move his feet before you begin working with him. Positioning the horse where you want him *before* you start the Technique accomplishes this.

2. Start with *Lateral Cervical Flexion*.
You will have already done the *Lateral Cervical Flexion Technique* and *Released the Scapula* (pp. 33 and 62). You can loosen and relax the neck before starting this Technique by doing a little bit of light lateral cervical flexion, working your way gently down the vertebrae of the neck to the scapula area.

QUICK OVERVIEW: Step-by-Step

TECHNIQUE 3: UNDER THE SCAPULA—C7-T1 JUNCTION RELEASE

Step 1. Stand at the horse's left shoulder with enough room to bring his nose around. Place your left leg a little behind you.

Step 2. Put your left hand gently on his nose and place the back of the right hand against his lower neck, a little higher up toward the withers, pointing down (Fig. 6.33 A).

Step 3. Make your right hand hard, gently increase pressure against the neck with the back of your hand, and find the fold of muscle in front of the scapula (B).

Step 4. Slide your hand down the underside of the muscle *very slowly*, watching the horse's eye, and feeling for the horse to tense (C).

Step 5. Shift the horse's weight gently to the opposite leg when you reach the area

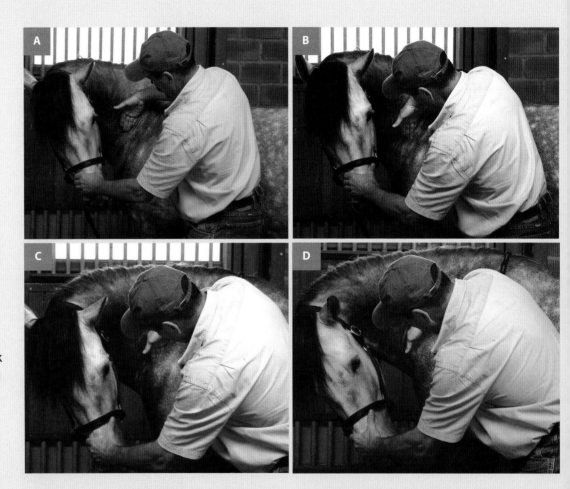

of the lower vertebra of the *Cervical-Thoracic Junction,* or when you feel the *brachiocephalic* muscle release. Use your weight to get him to slightly relax the near leg (D).

Step 6. Continue pushing your hand down through the muscle, out the bottom.

Step 7. Step back and see what he has to say.

3. Position yourself.

Stand as in figure 6.33 A with one hand lightly on the nose and the back of your other hand against the neck in front of the scapula.

Begin with your hand a little higher up toward to the withers of the horse to give you room to search for a fold in the muscle. Keep the flat of the back of your hand against the side of the horse's neck. You will need to have your fingers pointing toward the ground, and your elbow pointing somewhat in the air, as shown.

Stand far enough back toward the shoulder to give yourself room to bring his head around. It also helps to have your left hind leg a little out behind you so that you will be able to push against the horse's neck with your right (diagonal) hand.

4. Find a comfortable position for the horse's nose.

Gently bring the horse's nose toward you to relax the neck. Keep your nose hand soft so the horse stays soft and bring it around to a point where he is comfortable. Watch his eyes as you do this. Usually his eyes will soften or he will blink when his head is at a comfortable position. Some horses are comfortable with their heads more toward the front, others more flexed. Feel for where they are most relaxed before you start.

5. Start to push down under the front of the scapula.

Apply gentle pressure with the back of your hand to the horse's neck to relax it, and gently push downward, under the muscle, toward the ground. Keep the back of your hand against the neck, and keep your fingers as stiff as possible. Use enough pressure—*lemon*—so that you can get your fingertips under the fold of muscle in front of the scapula. It may take a little searching to find the right fold of muscle: It's a little deeper than you think.

Try not to grab with your fingers, instead make your hand rigid like a board and try to slide under the edge of the muscle as you slide your hand down toward the ground (fig. 6.34).

Go very slowly and very deep, and if you even sense the horse's head start to rise or his muscles start to tense, then stop moving your hand and *hold what you have* for just a few seconds, then continue on. Watch his eye as your hand goes down: If he blinks, hold for a second to give him time to relax, then move ahead.

Keep your nose hand as soft as possible (fig. 6.35). If you grab the nose, the horse will tense up. You want to stay below the horse's tensing threshold but still make forward progress.

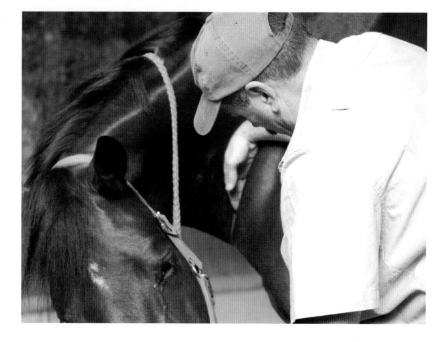

6.34 The trick is to keep your hand flat against the neck and your fingers stiff like a board. Take it slowly so that the horse can relax the muscle as you go.

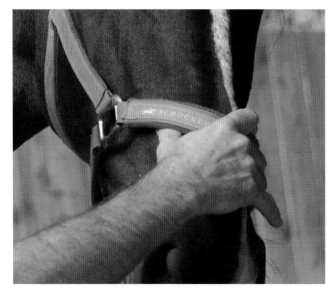

6.35 Keep your hand that is on the horse's nose as soft as possible.

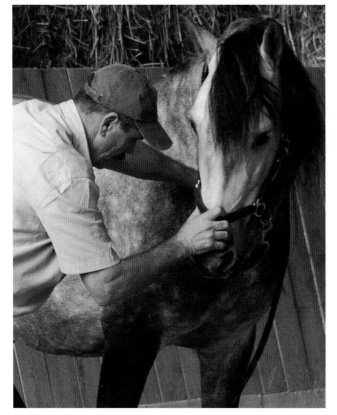

6.36 Lean slightly into the horse to ask him to shift his weight.

If the horse starts to raise his head or take it away, yield slightly to "keep him in the neighborhood." You can create a firm boundary but remember to soften and yield the instant he softens and yields. If you find yourself bracing against the horse, it isn't working.

6. Continue sliding your hand down.

Slide on down under the muscle in front of the shoulder. Stop when you run out of horse and your hand comes out the bottom. You will often feel the muscle there relax—the lower end of the *brachiocephalic*. This is close to where it inserts on the forearm of the horse. When you feel this muscle "let go," the horse has released major tension there.

7. Ask the horse to shift his weight slightly to the opposite leg.

As you get under the muscle and your hand slides down to about where the back of your hand is against the lower vertebra, lean slightly into the horse to ask him to shift his weight to the opposite leg (fig. 6.36). When he relaxes the leg nearest you he will release tension in this joint.

Tips

- Remember to keep your neck hand hard and proceed gently, staying "under the horse's radar".

- Keep your nose hand *soft* whenever the horse is soft.

- Anticipate when the horse begins to tense, and stop pushing down. Hold what you've got until the horse relaxes a bit, then continue on down.

■ Use your weight to ask the horse to shift his weight slightly to the opposite leg.

Note: With all of these Techniques, when you can anticipate even the slightest tensing or resistance before it happens, yield to it the slightest bit, then move immediately forward through it, the horse will release the resistance. Even if you sense some resistance and you're not really sure it's there, soften slightly then move forward.

Watch the horse's eye closely as you move forward, and consciously keep your hands as soft as you can as you work. If you feel or anticipate tensing, soften before the horse braces. Then gently move ahead with what you were doing. You will physically feel the resistance let go as the horse moves through it. When you come back afterward and ask the horse to move through it again, the resistance will be gone or there will be an improvement. Paying attention to this will help you through many difficulties with the horse.

What Ifs?

■ *What if the horse throws his head?*

There are a couple of reasons for this: One is that he is sore in the area where you are placing your hand (withers and lower neck). The first thing to do is soften both of your hands, but don't let go, or the horse will figure this out.

Another reason is because he may be a dominant horse and doesn't want a hand on his nose.

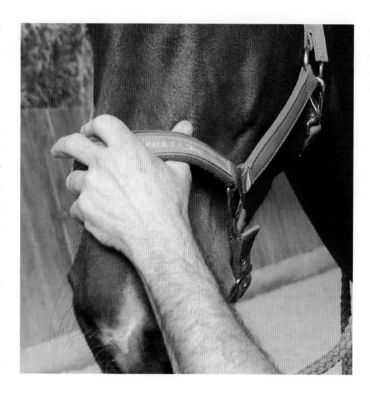

6.37 Slip your thumb and forefinger under and over the noseband.

This happens, especially with young horses, and even more with stallions. You can be firm to try to get the horse to stop throwing your hand off but remember, if he yields to your asking, you also have to yield immediately. Those are the rules!

If the horse keeps throwing his head, you can either train him to stop (although in most cases it is counterproductive) or switch your hand to his noseband, which usually works. These type of horses usually just want your hand off their nose but will tolerate the noseband).

Sometimes you can just let him throw his nose in the air a few times so that he feels like he's done something, then continue on.

Keep your hand resting lightly on the noseband. Slipping your thumb and forefinger under and over the noseband (as you learned during *lat-*

eral flexion) helps you to keep a light grip without bracing (fig. 6.37).

In any case, if you find yourself bracing against the horse, it isn't working.

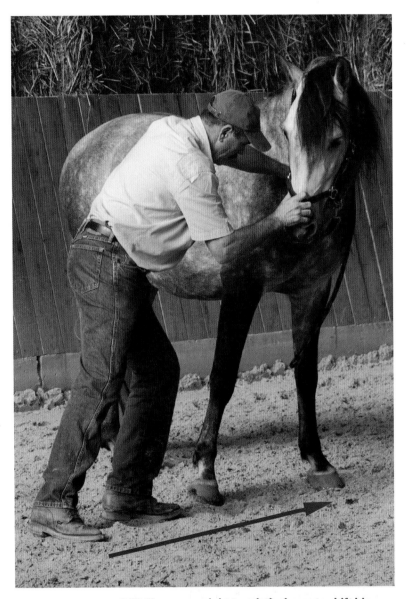

6.38 Use your weight to ask the horse to shift his weight slightly to the opposite leg.

■ *What if the horse moves his hind end around away from me and we keep going in circles?*

This is where your leg behind you comes in handy because you can use your weight to ask him to step away with the front legs each time he takes a step (fig. 6.38).

This will accomplish two things:

1. Each time he steps laterally while you have pressure on the lower neck, it will move this junction and release tension in it. You turn his walking away from you to your advantage, for the horse, too. Every step he takes, push hard—*lime* pressure—against his neck to get him to step laterally. You can push with your nose hand to help this. Just remember to soften each step as the horse's near leg steps back toward you in order to allow the horse to relax and release each step. When your timing is on, it almost turns into a dance.

2. Each time he steps away he will also get nearer to the wall where, if you don't want to dance, he will run out of room and let you finish running your hand under the muscle.

■ *What if my hand just won't go under the muscle, or it keeps "popping out" at a certain point?*

Continue, with the back of your hand against the lower neck on the outside of the muscle, to ask the horse to shift weight to the opposite leg and relax the near leg as much as possible (fig. 6.39). This will also release tension in the junction. This is a little bit of a balancing act and it may take a few times for *your* muscles to get attuned to what you're doing.

Some horses are too tight here to be able to

get under the muscle in one session, or even at all. Older horses, especially, can be so tight that it is hard to get completely under their muscle. However, you are only looking for an improvement each step of the way, and if you do the Technique without getting under the muscle—and step back to see what the horse has to say—he will usually tell you "That feels good!"

If you have trouble with this, do a couple *Scapula Releases* and go back and forth between Techniques a bit. Each time you will feel a little improvement.

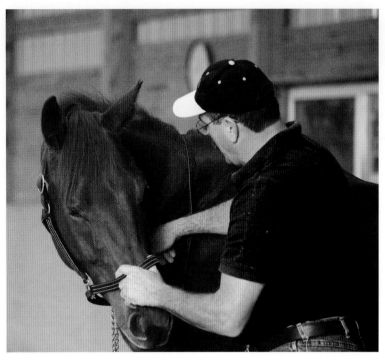

6.39 Shift the horse's weight to the opposite leg with your hand against the lower neck, on top of the muscle. You can see it more clearly in this photograph.

■ *What if he lowers his head to the ground?*

Most of the time this is a good thing, because the horse is relaxing that muscle, thus making it easier for you and him. Let him put his head where it is most comfortable. If he is lowering his head to try to evade what you are doing, you can ask him to bring it back up.

■ *What if he brings his head all the way around to touch his flank?*

He may be evading having you do the Technique, or he may think that's what you're asking him to do. In either case, push his head gently back toward the front a bit, wait until he relaxes, than start again.

Tip

■ With all of these Techniques, don't doubt your success or the effect they are having on the horse. If you feel that nothing is happening, come back the next day and try it again and you'll find that nine times out of ten, there will be an improvement in movement and the horse's ability to do the Technique. Many times you'll also find an improvement in relaxation and the horse's attitude. This is because he is often naturally uncomfortable showing the releases. It may also take a little time for the horse to feel that something has loosened up.

I constantly tell my students, if you're going to doubt anything, "Doubt the doubt!"

Technique 4:
WITHERS CHECK AND RELEASE (WITHERS WIGGLE)

Before You Begin

GOAL: In a relaxed state, to provide micro-movement of thoracic vertebrae beneath the scapula, through gentle movement of the withers to which they are attached (see the anatomy below).

RESULT: This subtle Technique releases deep-seated tension in largely inaccessible muscles surrounding the thoracic vertebrae beneath the scapula. Release of this tension further improves suspension, extension and fluidity of movement in the front end, and comfort and mobility in and behind the withers themselves.

WHERE YOU WORK—ANATOMY

Think of the withers as extensions (the *dorsal spinous processes*) of the thoracic vertebrae of the trunk. Generally the fourth or fifth (T4, T5) through the eighth or ninth (T8, T9) processes, depending on

the horse, are the ones you can feel. You can use these extensions to ask for gentle movement in vertebrae buried deep in the trunk of the horse that you would normally not be able to access.

RELEASING TENSION: THE EFFECTS

I compare the effect that tension in this part of the spine has on the horse's movement to how we as humans feel when we have knots or tension deep between our shoulder blades. The difference here is that with the horse, it is *very* deep.

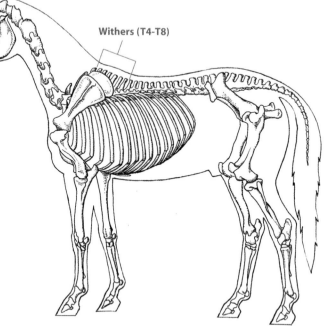

Withers (T4–T8)

6.40 The withers are the spinous processes of thoracic vertebrae T4 through T8

QUICK OVERVIEW: Step-by-Step

TECHNIQUE 4: WITHERS CHECK AND RELEASE (WITHERS WIGGLE)

Step 1. Place your fingers on a spinous process (wither), watching the horse's eyes (A).

Step 2. Wiggle it side to side.

Step 3. Stop.

Step 4. Watch for blink.

Step 5. Move to another spinous process (B).

Step 6. Wiggle, wiggle, wiggle.

Step 7. Stop.

Step 8. Watch for blink.

Step 9. Move to another spinous process (C).

Step 10. And so on.

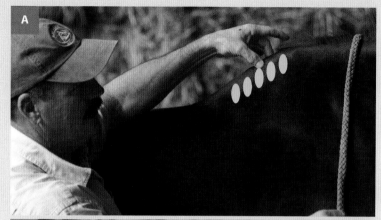

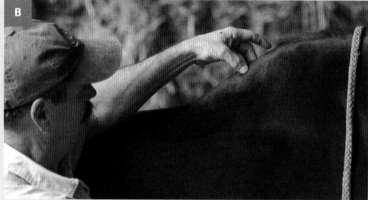

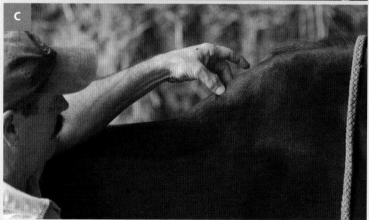

You can see by release responses how profound this simple yet deep Technique can be in some horses. Often, the effect that tension here has on performance isn't even noticed until it is released.

Technique 4 in More Detail

This is a very simple Technique but however lightly you think you are performing it, you can probably do it *lighter*, and with better results:

1. Position yourself.
Face the horse's withers so that you can watch the eyes. With just your fingers, lightly hold the first bump—spinous process—that you can feel. *Very gently* (*egg yolk* or *very soft grape* pressure) wiggle the spinous process (wither) from side to side, closely watching the eye for the slightest blink. If there is tension in that vertebra, the eye will twitch. If the eye blinks, wiggle again. Continue this and eventually the horse will start to release more tension and give you larger release responses. These will vary from licking and chewing, to repeated yawing. You may be surprised how much tension the horse can release with this easy exercise.

Watching for subtle responses to this movement indicates whether there is tension and when it has been released.

2. Work lightly.
Gentle movement of a joint or junction in its relaxed state releases tension in that joint or junction. There is so much muscle and structure around these vertebrae that the horse can easily block any attempt to wiggle them from the withers. However, you go so lightly that the horse cannot guard against it. Even the slightest movement of a vertebra in a relaxed state will release tension in the joint. If you don't believe me, try it and ask the horse.

3. Wiggle, wiggle, stop.
Because the horse can easily block out any movement here, it works well to wiggle the withers in small increments: wiggle, wiggle, stop (watch for blink); wiggle, wiggle, stop (watch for blink); wiggle, wiggle, stop (watch for blink). By stopping frequently, the horse's body doesn't have the chance to get used to the wiggle and block it out.

You can wiggle more than one spinous process at a time using the heel of your hand and more than one finger. However, the pressure rule remains the same—*grape* to *egg yolk* pressure.

Tip

- Don't think of this so much as a movement or a wiggle but as a signal you're sending to the thoracic vertebra through its spinous process (wither) to release tension. This Technique is as simple as that.

What Ifs?

- ***What if nothing happens?***

There may be nothing there to release so the horse gives you no response. However, it is worth spending half a minute or so experimenting, first with less pressure. Do this for about 30 seconds:

wiggle, wiggle, stop (watch for blink); wiggle, wiggle, stop (watch for blink). Horses can be very good at blocking you out, but if you go long enough and soft enough, you'll be surprised at what the horse will give you. You may try with a little more pressure. Spend half a minute. The horse may respond to this. The horse ultimately has the say on what level of pressure to use. Go by his responses.

If you get no response after half a minute, move on to the next Technique.

Note: *Often, it is after you step back or walk away that the horse will show you the release. It's just the way some horses are programmed.*

▪ *How often should I do this?*

You can't do any harm with this Technique but if you do it every day, at some point the horse will stop responding. Either there will be no more tension to release, or the horse will get used to it.

I often do it while standing and talking to a horse owner, to check the withers and just to give me something to do. It doesn't mean I'm not paying attention to what the owner has to say, but I'm also paying attention to the horse.

Just check your horse's withers every once in a while, or do it as long as the horse responds.

▪ *How long should I do this on one wither before moving to another one?*

It works well to do a couple of wiggles going down the line on each spinous process and see which ones the horse responds to. Then go back and do a little on each one again. If you do the same thing over and over, or for too long, the horse's body gets used to it and sometimes stops responding.

7

CHAPTER 7

The Hind End

Techniques 1 & 2:

- ■ **WORKING THE HIND END— *FROM THE TOP***
- ■ **WORKING THE HIND END— *FROM THE BOTTOM***

Before You Begin

This chapter is a little like the muscles and structure of the hind end itself—large and sometimes

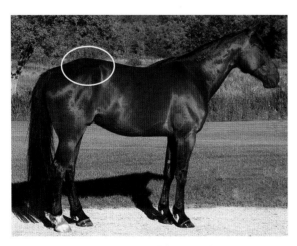

7.1 Key Junction 3: The Sacroiliac Junction.

a little intimidating. First you will find a detailed description of that anatomy and an explanation of how tension here can affect performance. However, as large and complicated as all of this might seem, all you *really* need in order to work on the hind end is a simple understanding of the Techniques, and the willingness to slow down and follow the horse's responses. There are two basic *Hind End Techniques* to use:

The first Technique, *Working the Hind End from the Top,* uses *Release Points* located higher up on the body to encourage relaxation of muscles surrounding this key junction.

The second, *Working the Hind End from the Bottom,* involves using the hind legs to release tension in this key junction with releases similar to those used on the front end. This Technique is in two parts: a) *Releasing the Hind Leg—Down and Forward* and b) *Releasing the Hind—Down and Back.* Both of these Techniques are described in detail ahead.

As mentioned above, the muscles and structures of the *hind end* are much bigger than those you have been working with on the *front end.* The hind end is the "motor" of the horse and the forces transferred from the powerful hind legs through the complex structure of the pelvis, sacrum, and sacroiliac to the body are immense. The tension that builds up here can be deep-rooted and may have been building up over a period of time.

Many performance issues have their origin in restrictions in the hind end.

It will be important to slow down and give the horse time to release tension in the hind end. This makes sense as the muscles are larger and have less movement and articulation than the muscles of the front end. However, you will also see that the releases you get—with surprisingly little force—and the responses the horse gives you when you get the releases, are large and even profound.

Let's get started by taking a look at the anatomy involved.

WHERE YOU WORK—ANATOMY

Skeletal Structure of the Hind End

The Sacroiliac Joint

Pelvis: The pelvis is a large framework that girdles the spinal column of the hind end. It anchors muscles that are essential in locomotion and the transference of force from the hind limbs to the body, and it protects organs in the abdominal cavity (figs. 7. 3 and 7.8, p. 109).

Ilium: The ilium is the largest part of the pelvis and forms the two top parts on each side (fig. 7.8). To locate the tips of the ilium, stand at the tail (of a relatively short horse) facing forward, put your arms in front of you, and place your fingertips on the two bones at the *highest* point, or *top* of the croup. You can feel the tops of its two "wings" if you run your fingertips from side to side across the *highest* point of the hindquarters.

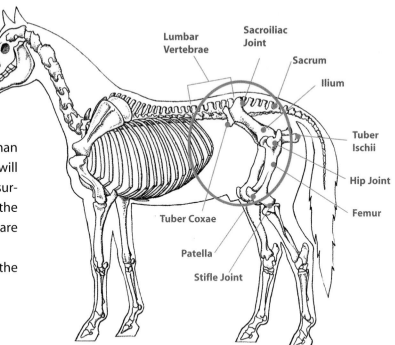

7.2 The sacroiliac area.

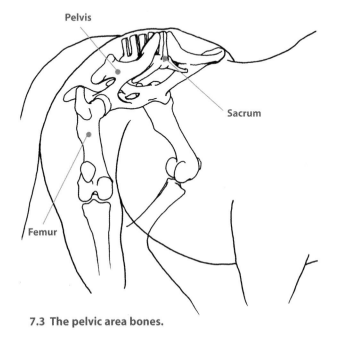

7.3 The pelvic area bones.

These are called the *tuber sacrales* of the ilium (see fig. 7.8 again).

Tuber coxae: These are the two widest points of the pelvis. To locate them stand at the tail (of a relatively thin horse) facing forward, put your arms in front of you and place your fingertips on the two bones at the *widest* part of the hip, also called the "points of the hip."

Sacrum: The sacrum is a solid bone made up of the last five vertebrae of the spinal column before the tail. They are fused together into one triangle-shaped bone pointing toward the tail (figs. 7.3 and 7.8).

Sacroiliac joint: This is where the sacrum joins with the ilium (sacroiliac). The two flat surfaces of the ilium lie on top of each of the wings of the sacrum. Between them is the sacroiliac ligament, a large flat ligament that connects them to form the sacroiliac joint (figs. 7.3 and 7.8).

Hip joint and femur: The hip joint is the socket where the thigh bone (femur) connects to the

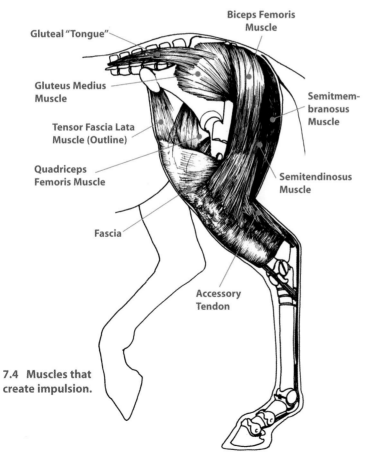

Gluteal "Tongue"

Biceps Femoris
Muscle

Gluteus Medius
Muscle

Tensor Fascia Lata
Muscle (Outline)

Semitmem-
branosus
Muscle

Quadriceps
Femoris Muscle

Semitendinosus
Muscle

Fascia

Accessory
Tendon

7.4 Muscles that create impulsion.

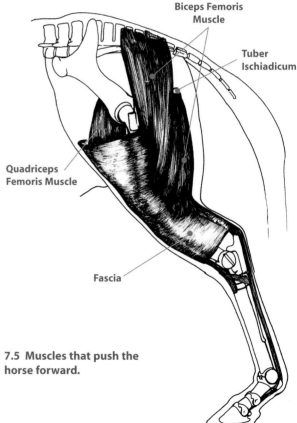

Biceps Femoris
Muscle

Tuber
Ischiadicum

Quadriceps
Femoris Muscle

Fascia

7.5 Muscles that push the horse forward.

pelvis at the hip joint, or acetabulum (figs. 7.3 and 7.8). Stress can accumulate here as muscle spasms. These spasms are an indication of excessive tension in the middle gluteal muscles.

The hip joint is also a *Release Point* for tension in the lumbar area where the middle gluteal muscle originates (fig. 7.4).

Major Muscles of the Hind End

Middle gluteal muscle: The largest of the gluteal muscles—the *middle gluteal*—is one of the major driving muscles of the horse (see *gluteus medius,* fig. 7.4). It originates in the lumbar region (see gluteal "tongue", fig. 7.4), and inserts (ends) at the hip joint on the *greater trochanter* of the femur. Releasing tension in this muscle also helps to release tension in the lumbar spine.

Hamstring muscle: This group of important driving muscles *(biceps femoris, semitendinosus, semimembranosus)* anchor on the sacrum (fig. 7.5) and drive the body forward. If they accumulate tension and become restricted they can put excessive and imbalanced tension on the sacrum and *Sacroiliac Junction.*

Psoas: These unseen muscles are major stabilizers of the horse's lumbar and pelvic area (fig. 7.6). They also flex the hip and are involved in the transference of power from the hind limbs to the trunk. They connect the underside of the lumbar with pelvis and hind legs.

Groin muscles: Groin muscles are very important in that once injured, they require a while to heal (fig.

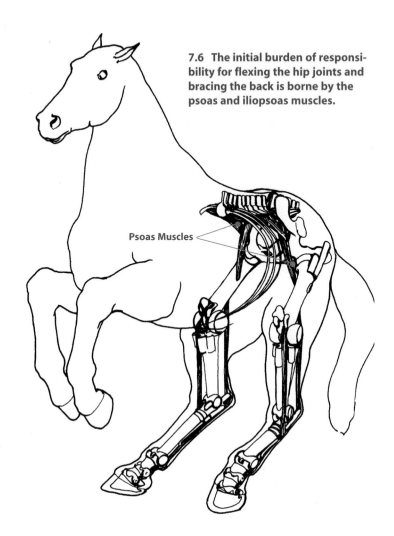

7.6 The initial burden of responsibility for flexing the hip joints and bracing the back is borne by the psoas and iliopsoas muscles.

Psoas Muscles

7.7). I have found that they are often associated with tension in the stifles.

Major Ligaments of the Hind End

Sacroiliac ligaments: These broad bands of strong fibrous connective tissue work to hold the *sacrum* and the *ilium* together. The inner sacroiliac ligament lies in the flat narrow space between the ilium and the sacrum, while the dorsal sacroiliac ligament lies behind and on top (see fig. 7.8, p. 109).

As with most ligaments, these are designed to stabilize and hold joints together and don't have much stretch and flexibility. The sacroiliac *joint* isn't what you would call an articulating joint. However, it is very large and when tension accumulates on it the whole area is affected.

Note: *When tension on the sacroiliac joint is released via sacroiliac ligaments, tension in the major muscles of the hind end also releases.*

Sacrotuberous ligament: This is a broad, flat ligament that connects under the tail at the sacrum on the top end, to the *ischium* (butt bone) on the pelvis at the bottom end. Tension on this ligament puts tension or "torque" on the sacrum and on the sacroiliac joint.

THE IMPORTANCE OF THE SACRUM AND SACROILIAC JOINT

Tension on any of the three key junctions of *Poll-Atlas; Neck-Shoulder-Withers;* and *Sacroiliac Joint (sacrum-ilium)* can cause excessive tension to accumulate in respective major muscles and connective tissue. In addition, excessive unilateral (one-sided) use of these muscles will create a unilateral imbalance of tension on these junctions.

The sacrum is an important anchoring point in the transference of driving forces from the hind limbs to the body. If tension accumulates in the muscles that pull on the

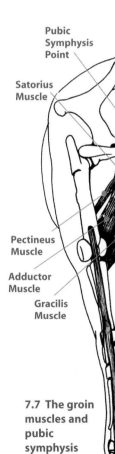

Pubic Symphysis Point

Satorius Muscle

Pectineus Muscle

Adductor Muscle

Gracilis Muscle

7.7 The groin muscles and pubic symphysis point.

sacrum, the sacroiliac joint can become restricted, tight or "stuck."

This tension or restriction can have a negative effect on the muscles of the hind end that makes it difficult for those muscles to let go.

Releasing tension on the sacrum helps to release tension in the muscles of the hind end. Tension can accumulate on the sacrum from:

1. *Normal work and conditioning.* Given the size of the muscles and the amount of force that is transferred via these muscles from the hind limbs to the body, it is no surprise that tension builds up here.

2. *Over-conditioning and training.* When one group of muscles is consistently asked to do an excess of work before other, supporting muscles are fit to support that work, the tension that builds up between those interdependent groups will not be balanced or distributed evenly.

3. *The natural predisposition of the horse to favor one side over the other.*

As with humans, most horses have a stronger or predominant side and may be more comfortable using one particular side or diagonal. This can naturally create unilateral tension on muscles that pull on major components of the hind end such as the sacrum or *Sacroiliac Junction,* and lumbar spine or lower back.

The added effects of over-conditioning or training can increase this imbalance.

4. *Compensation for soreness or restriction in other areas of the body.* As one part of the horse involved in a certain movement becomes sore or restricted and begins to function less efficiently, other parts have to take some of the load.

This can happen from front to back, for example: As components of the hind end become sore, restricted, or don't function properly, the horse tends to go more on the forehand or use muscles of the front end to pull himself along.

Compensation can also occur by area. For example, if the *Sacroiliac Junction* and the lumbar area of the horse are restricted and not functioning properly, then more load will be put on the *muscles, tendons, and ligaments* of the hind legs.

This is explained in more detail in chapter 9 (p. 160).

5. *Moving in unnatural or stressed positions that don't allow the body to work as a whole.* This can lead to excessive and unbalanced tension in different areas of the horse.

RELEASING TENSION: THE EFFECTS

Hind End Tension on the Horse's Back

Back pain or discomfort is one of the most common complaints horse owners and trainers bring to the table. You've already learned that there is a connection between tension in the poll and tension in the back. There is also a connection between tension in the *hind end* and tension in the back.

The forces generated by a horse's hind end are immense. In an *unrestricted* horse these forces travel through the spine to the front end. When horses become *restricted* in the sacroiliac junction due to any combination of factors rather than the forces

moving smoothly forward through the body, then the brunt of the load is taken by the sacroiliac joint, lumbar spine and *Sacrolumbar Junction.* The lower back becomes stressed and painful, the horse compensates for the pain, and a cycle of back pain and negative self-carriage begins.

Techniques to release tension on the sacrum start the process of breaking this cycle. That is, of course, if the issues that contributed to the hind-end problem or back problem to begin with have been resolved.

Hind End Tension on the Front End

You will notice while working on the poll that often a hind leg will buckle, relax, wobble, or the horse may stomp or kick out with a hind foot. This

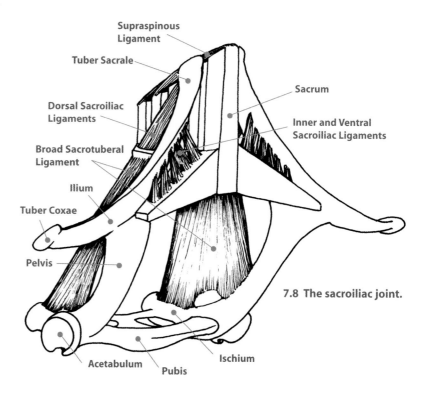

7.8 The sacroiliac joint.

is a *direct, observable connection* between release of tension in the atlas, and release of tension in the sacrum and gluteal muscles.

There is also a connection between the release of tension in the lower neck *(C7-T1 Junction),* and signs of release of tension in the hind end. The most obvious connections are below:

■ One of the most important muscles involved in locomotion of the horse, the *longissimus dorsi,* anchors in the lower neck at C5, 6, and 7, and at the other end at the pelvis (fig. 7.9).

■ The *nuchal* and *supraspinous* ligament system forms one long connection from the top of the poll to the top of the withers and spine, to the sacrum (see fig. 5.4, p. 35).

Longissimus Muscle
(cervical part)

Iliocostalis Muscle

Longissimus
Muscle (lumbar
and thoracic part)

Psoas Group
of Muscles

Longissimus Muscle
(parts to the first neck
vertebrae and skull)

**7.9 Muscular con-
nection between
front and hind end.**

■ A connection from the front end of the horse to the pelvis via a lower contraction system of abdominal muscles balances out the back connections above, and is an important player in self carriage and locomotion in the horse.

■ And finally, a neurological connection will become clear when you are using the Techniques to release tension in the atlas and observe the hind end begin to relax and wobble. You will find that spasms in the gluteal muscles at the hip joint often relax or even disappear once the atlas is released!

These examples give an idea of how the different mechanisms of the body are interconnected and interdependent, and how abnormal tension that develops in any one part of the body can affect other parts of the body and their functions.

The Atlas-Sacrum Connection

Note: When discomfort shows up anywhere in the body it is reflected by tension in the poll and atlas!

When you release tension in the poll, you begin the process of release in the sacrum and the hind end. And when you release tension in the sacrum, you begin the process of release in the poll. Don't ask me how this works: It's a mystery. But it works!

The Effects of Hind End Tension on Overall Performance

Some of the more observable performance issues

that can be the result of excessive or unbalanced tension in the hind end are:

- Lack of impulsion, meaning the horse's pushing power or thrust is limited.

- Inability to round, step under, or develop "positive" self-carriage. (Note: Flexibility of the lumbar area is key and allows the horse to twist and be able to tilt the pelvis and step under.)

Performance problems become even more apparent when excessive tension develops unilaterally, meaning more to one side than the other. Some signs of this are:

- Refusal to put more weight on a particular hind limb, and resistance to moving on a circle in one direction or the other.

- Inability or unwillingness to canter on a particular lead.

- Refusal or unwillingness to pick up the foot for cleaning or the farrier (ruling out neurological conditions such as stringhalt, see p. 136).

- The horse may appear unsound with no apparent cause.

- Or, he may seem imbalanced or excessive tension allowed to remain for too long leads to lameness issues in the joints, tendons and ligaments of the hind limbs.

Note: *It's important that a veterinarian is consulted to eliminate the possibility of an injury that may be* contributing to any of these performance issues. However, once an injury or veterinary issue has been ruled out, you can explore whether excessive or imbalanced tension might be a contributor by simply beginning to release tension in your horse, then see if there is an improvement. If there is, do more!

Technique 1:
WORKING THE HIND END— *FROM THE TOP*

Let's begin releasing tension in this area with *Technique 1: Working the Hind End—From the Top.*

GOAL: To soften or relax the hind end and encourage the horse to relax each leg and drop the pelvis beyond the normal *relaxed* range of movement, by using light touch on certain points on the hind end.

RESULT: Allows the horse to release tension in the sacroiliac joint, lumbar area and sacrolumbar junction. The farther the leg and pelvis drop to one side, the more of a relaxed "twist" you will get in the lumbar vertebrae, helping to release tension in the muscles of the lower back.

HOW IT WORKS

This soft Technique involves using different levels of light touch on certain *Release Points* on the hind end. Bringing the horse's attention to these points sends signals to the horse's nervous system to relax tension in the pelvis and sacrum. When this happens, the horse displays normal release responses and eventually drops the pelvis on one side, then drops it on the other.

When working the hind end *From the Top* you follow the responses just as you did with the *Bladder Meridian Technique*. Rather than using pressure, you are in a sense sending neurological signals to the horse's body to relax and release tension.

The levels of touch you use on these points vary from very light, *air gap,* to medium, *grape/lemon* (see p. 6 for touch pressures).

The key qualities you need for success are: softness, patience, and ability to closely follow the responses of the horse to your touch.

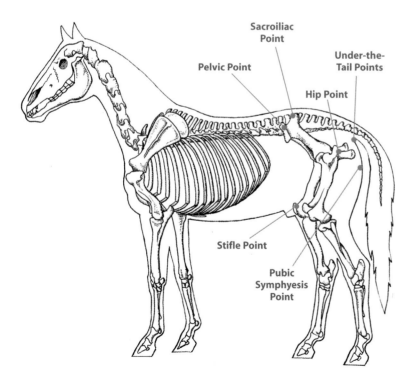

Sacroiliac Point

Pelvic Point

Under-the-Tail Points

Hip Point

Stifle Point

Pubic Symphyesis Point

7.10 **The six** *Release Points.*

Sound easy? It is. In fact it's much easier, simpler, and more effective than you might think.

Release Points to Use When Working *From the Top*

There are six *Release Points* that you'll use to ask the horse's nervous system to let go of tension in the sacrum and pelvis. Their general location is described below, but the most effective way to pinpoint them is to ask the horse exactly where they are by using air-gap touch to search for a subtle response such as a blink, twitch, or change of breath, similar to what you do with the *Bladder Meridian Technique* (Search, Response, Stay, Release!)

The six Release Points are:
1. The Sacrotuberous Ligament (Under-the-Tail) Points (2 of them).
2. The Sacroiliac Point (1).
3. The Hip Joint Point (2).
4. The Pelvic Points (2).
5. The Stifle Points (2).
6. The Pubic Symphysis (PS) Point (1).

HOW TO USE THE RELEASE POINTS

Unlike most of the Techniques I've presented so far, there really are no *step-by-step* instructions for using these *Release Points*, other than this one:

An *Under-the-Tail Point* is always the best place to start working *From the Top*. After that, the *Release Points* do not need to be used in any particular sequence. Pay attention and the horse and your intuition will guide you to the next point(s) to use.

This is, in a sense, an experiment or exploration to discover which *Release Points* work best on a particular horse. Every horse is different and responds differently to different points, depending on each individual horse's tension patterns.

Remember, the goal of using these points is to get the horse to relax and drop first one side of the pelvis and then the other. Each time this happens you continue using different points to encourage the pelvis to drop further.

Every time the horse relaxes and drops the pelvis beyond the previous normal *relaxed* range of movement, or point of restriction, it allows the sacroiliac joint to release more and more tension. It's actually all very simple once you get started.

HOW TO BEGIN

As a general rule we start on the *right* side of the hind end because, in most cases, the horse's left hind will be the tighter side.

Where you go *after* you've used the *Under-the-Tail Point* depends on what the horse does or tells you with his responses.

For example, if the horse drops a hip while you are focusing on any point, go to the "dropped" side and use the points there to encourage the horse to drop even further (fig. 7.11). If you are using a very light touch, the slightest blink or twitch will tell you that this is a good place to stay.

When the horse gets tired of standing on that leg and shifts to the other, you can go to any of the points on the newly dropped side and encourage the pelvis to relax even further there.

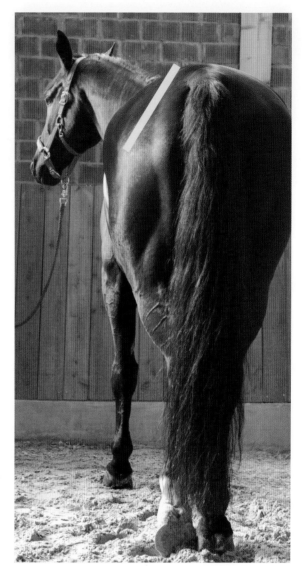

7.11 If the horse drops a hip while you are focusing on a point, go to the "dropped-hip" side and touch another Release Point to encourage more "drop."

Each time the pelvis drops on a side you will notice that it is a little lower than before. Also notice that there will be more and more of a relaxed twist in the lumbar area or lower back as tension "lets go" there. And you will sooner or later notice larger release responses, such as yawning or shaking the head, that go along with it.

KEYS TO SUCCESS

■ Don't have expectations or an agenda: Every horse responds differently to each *Release Point* depending on where he is holding his tension, his personality and body type.

■ Throw away the clock!

■ Don't think too much. Use your intuition when deciding whether to stay on a point until you get a (bigger) release or move on.

Intuition

What is intuition? *Merriam Webster* dictionary says, "...the power or faculty of attaining to direct knowledge or cognition without evident rational thought and inference..."

In other words: You are seeing subtle anomalies—or changes—in the horse that you are not consciously aware of when your analytical mind is in the way.

The more you quiet down and observe without analyzing, the more your intuition will kick in, the more subtle changes you will see, and the more effective your bodywork will be. Watching and waiting for the subtle responses from the horse is an effective way of quieting down. The rest comes naturally.

When you have slowed down, just look at the horse and do what comes next naturally. And don't worry too much about it. Your intuition will lead you to the next step. And the best part is that you can't really hurt the horse or do this wrong. You can only do good, or better.

■ Observe more, analyze less. Once you are "out of your mind," you will find your intuition kicking in more readily and you won't have to think so much about which point to go to next.

Safety Note: When you first start, be aware that the horse could be extremely sore or sensitive to any touch or pressure on any of these points. With this method you shouldn't be using enough pressure to cause any discomfort; however, the horse may still be surprised when you place a finger on a sensitive area or point. If you aren't sure, stand to the side and as far forward as possible, and always watch for a flattening of the ears anytime you approach a potentially sensitive area.

What follows are detailed descriptions of the locations of the six *Release Points* and tips on what levels of touch to use (or not use) along with possible sequences.

1. Sacrotuberous Ligament (Under-the-Tail, or UTP) Point

There are two of these points, one on the right and one on the left (figs. 7.12 A & B)

These points release tension on the sacro-tuberous ligaments where they attach in the area of the tail end of the sacrum. This point is the ideal place to begin work on the hind end when you've finished with the *Front End Techniques*. It begins the process of relaxing tension on the sacrum and on the whole horse. In addition, it begins the process of relaxing you after all the movement and sometimes strenuous activity involved in some of the *Front End Techniques*.

Tips

■ As mentioned at the beginning of this book, when you begin work on the horse you generally begin at the left front, which is often the easier side for the horse, then move to the right front, which is generally the tighter side, then move to the right hind, which is generally the easier side behind, then the left hind, which being the diagonal to the right front is generally the tighter side behind.

As a general rule, begin with the *right Under the-Tail Point*. If you find that the horse is uncomfortable with this, go to the left point.

To access the *right* point, position yourself at the *left* side of the horse's rump facing forward. Gently raise the tail, rest your right hand on the rump (fig. 7.13 A) and *softly* place your right thumb at the deepest point you are able to touch under the tail, a little off to the right, at about the one o'clock position on the "dial."

To access the *left* point, position yourself at the *right* side of the horse's rump facing forward. Gently raise the tail, rest

your right hand on the rump (fig. 7.13 B) and *softly* place your right thumb at the deepest point you are able to touch under the tail, a little off to the right, at about the eleven o'clock position on the "dial."

■ It's important to start with very light pressure on this point—literally between *air gap* and *egg yolk*.

■ It makes a big difference (to the horse) whether you are applying light touch with a *soft* hand, or light touch with a *hard* hand. *Consciously keep your hand soft while using these points.*

■ It isn't the pressure that releases this ligament—it's more that you are sending a "signal"

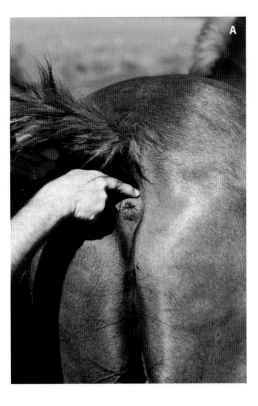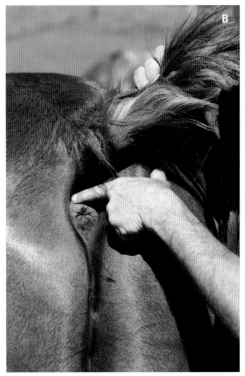

7.12 A & B The location of the right Under-the-Tail Point: one o'clock on the "dial" (A). The location of the left Under-the-Tail Point: eleven o'clock on the dial (B).

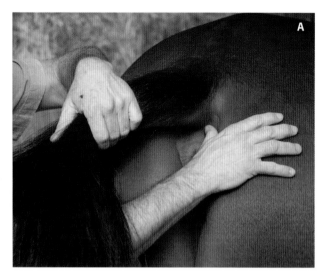 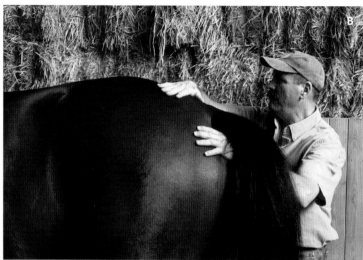

An Embarrassing Situation!

The Sacrotuberous Ligament Technique is actually known to human chiropractors as the "Logan Basic" maneuver. You should consider yourself lucky not to be a human chiropractor! It's strange enough to have someone walk by a stall and see you standing there with your thumb under the tail of the horse. Usually a comment such as, "Well, the tonsils seem to be okay!" or "Cough!" lightens up the atmosphere..

I was once at a hunter-jumper show when a trainer asked me to work on one of his client's horses. At one point while working on the front end the horse was asleep with his head up on my shoulder with my arms around his neck as I massaged the muscles behind the poll. The lady who owned the horse happened to walk by the stall at that moment, stopped briefly to watch and said, "Eew! That looks weird!"

I looked over the horse's neck at her and replied, "Wait 'till you see what happens at the other end!"

to the horse's nervous system. So wait for it to respond. Watch the horse's eyes: Blinks will tell you when the tension is letting go.

- It may take three seconds, 30 seconds, or 60 seconds; every horse is different. If after 30 seconds you get no response, adjust your (non-) pressure, or try slightly moving your thumb.

- Stay on this point until you get a release response. If you get no response, spend 60 to 90 seconds here before moving on. If you get no response it doesn't mean it isn't working: It may be that the horse is not letting you know he has released, or that there was no tension there to release. But if you stay long enough—and soft enough—on any point where there is tension, the horse's nervous system will *have* to release it.

- What to do with the other hand? You can rest it lightly on the SI (sacroiliac joint) while doing the *Under-the-Tail Points,* if you wish. This will help relax this area.

- When the horse clamps his tail down and is uncomfortable with this point, it is a sign that there could be tension in the sacrum, hamstrings, or both. When this happens, try sliding your hand farther down the tail and gently lifting it, waiting for the horse to relax it. Then it may be easier to sneak into the *Under-the-Tail Point.*

- You don't have to do both *Under the Tail Points* one after the other. Start with one and then follow the releases. Come back to the other point any time during the session or when you feel the time is right to begin working on the other side.

Safety Note: *Be very aware of the horse's reaction when first approaching these points. Go gently, and "watch the ears"! If they are pinned back, stop! Horses with extreme tension in the sacrum, hamstrings or groin can be VERY sensitive here. Don't just lift the tail and jab your fingers in there!*

If you are not sure, skip this Release Point until a later time. The horse may have relaxed enough to let you in there after he has released tension in the pelvis on other points. If there is any doubt at all, bypass this point. And, as an added safety precaution, you may want to place a couple of bales of hay

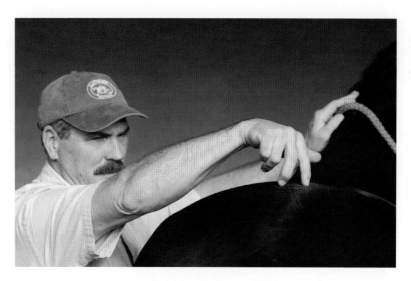

7.14 These two "bumps" are at the top of the sacroiliac joint. Search here for the horse's blink.

between you and the hind end before doing this.

2. Sacroiliac (SI) Point

This point is located in the area of the two *ilium* bones at the high point, or croup, of the hind end. This important point affects the large *sacroiliac joint* as the key junction of the pelvis and the sacrum (fig. 7.14). Using this point sends signals to the nervous system to help the sacroiliac joint release tension.

Tips

- Generally it is good to start by searching with *air-gap* pressure for the blink, letting the horse tell you *exactly* where to start.

- You can increase to *egg yolk* after the horse has dropped the hip to one side, encouraging him to drop even more. If you use too much pressure, the horse will be uncomfortable and let

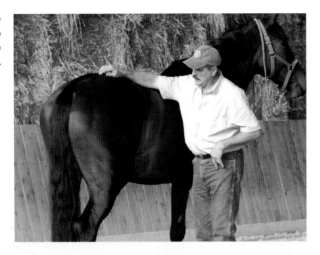

7.15 Move to the "dropped" side to encourage more release.

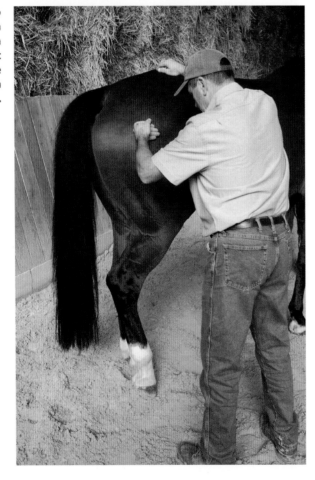

7.16 Use the Hip Joint Point in conjunction with the Sacroiliac Point to encourage more relaxation and release.

you know by putting weight back on the leg, or stepping away.

■ If the horse has dropped a hip while on any point, it helps to go to the *Sacroiliac Point on the side that has dropped* (fig. 7.15). Searching for a blink from the horse, place your fingertips about an inch off the centerline, on the bone *(tuber sacral)*. This encourages the horse's body to relax this joint and drop the hip even further.

■ Try using this point in conjunction with the *Hip Joint Point* to encourage more relaxation and release (fig. 7.16).

■ If you think the horse is not responding, step away and give him time to "feel" what is going on. When you step away, step *way* away. Avoid the temptation to stay close and pet him. He may need space to release. With some horses, it's not until you leave the stall entirely that they will "let go."

3. The Hip Joint Point

This point is located near the top and a little forward of the poverty groove, or delineation between the hamstring muscles (fig. 7.17). On horses with less "meat" you can feel a slight "bump and hollow" here. On others you may feel nothing. Search for the blink.

The middle gluteal *(gluteus medius)* muscle, which originates in the lower back (lumbar area), inserts here at the hip joint. This is one of the horse's main driving muscles and can spasm at its insertion point. When you relax this muscle it helps to relieve tension in the lower back.

Tips

■ You can use *air gap* to search for the exact spot. Start lightly and be patient. Often the horse will drop the hip just from this light touch.

■ If you feel that the horse has relaxed but has not yet dropped the hip, you can slowly apply gentle pressure against the hip at this point (see fig. 7.16) to encourage the horse to shift weight to the opposite leg and relax the near leg. Increase to *lemon pressure,* if needed. When the horse steps sideways, lighten the pressure immediately. When he puts weight back on the leg, apply more pressure until he stands still with the weight on the opposite leg.

4. The Pelvic Point

There are two bony protrusions on each side at the widest part of the pelvis. There is actually a bony ridge about 4 or 5 inches long that runs diagonally forward and downward. It is at the lower point on the underside of this bony ridge that you will find your *Pelvic Point.*

There are muscle and fascial attachments here that make this a very powerful point for releasing tension in the entire hind end in some horses. It is

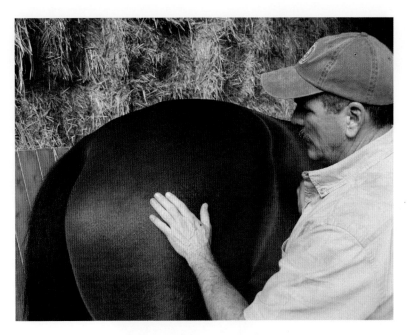

7.17 Search for the "blink" in this area to find the exact spot.

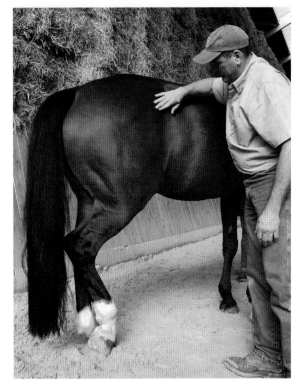

7.18 Search with very light pressure for the slightest blink on this point.

also a point that in my experience often correlates to tension or soreness in the stifles.

Tips

- Search with very light pressure (barely touching the tips of the hairs) for the slightest blink (fig. 7.18).

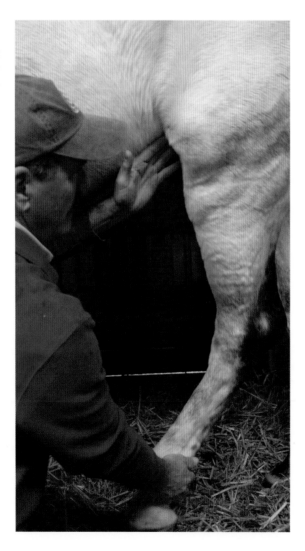

7.19 Use the Stifle Point to encourage the stifle to relax even more to the outside.

- This point is super-sensitive. Anything more than the lightest *air-gap* pressure will cause the horse to block this point out. You should almost be touching only one hair at a time here with the tip of one finger.

- Not all horses will be responsive to this point, but once you get a blink, be patient and stay (lightly) on the point. When you think you have waited long enough, wait just a little longer. You may be surprised when the hip suddenly drops.

Safety Note: Some horses, especially mares, can be very sensitive at the Pelvic Point or in the area of the flank and abdominals. Watch the ears! If they flatten back, STOP. Be sure that before you go to this area you have already touched the horse's flank and he is comfortable with you there.

5. The Stifle Point

This point is located in a soft indentation on the inside of the horse's upper leg in the stifle area. There is a bony protrusion just inside the stifle. The *Stifle Point* is behind this bony protuberance at the top of the tibia.

Tight groin muscles can put tension on the stifle. Horses that are tight in the forward part of the groin will have difficulty relaxing the stifle outward.

This point has the effect of relaxing the muscles that pull on the stifle. This includes the groin muscles, as well as deeper muscles of the hind end. By releasing tension here you are helping the stifle to stay healthy (and happy).

Tips

- Search with *air-gap* pressure to get the blink. Stay lightly with this pressure for at least a half a minute, waiting for further responses.

- Horses with sore stifles will often give large responses to this point.

- Once the hip has dropped this point works well to encourage the stifle to relax and "fall out" even more to the outside (fig. 7.19).

- Once the horse's leg is relaxed and he is resting it forward, place your hand gently on his hock and wiggle gently on the leg. Relaxed wiggling helps the relaxation and release process. If you wiggle too hard the horse will let you know by tensing up or putting weight on the leg.

- Using the "following the blink" method, you can search for points anywhere on the stifle, on the inside or the outside, that are holding tension.

Safety Note: *If the horse is sensitive or sore in the stifle, groin, or even the flank, he may flinch or kick if touched carelessly there (fig. 7.20 A). Watch the ears AND the leg. Stand as far forward toward the withers as possible when first touching the flank, or when placing your hand inside the hind leg.*

Begin by placing your hand down near the hock and gently slide up the outside, and then the inside of the stifle (fig. 7.20 B). Make sure the horse is not sensitive on the flanks before doing this. If there is any doubt, as with the other points, come back to this after the horse has released tension from other points, or skip this point altogether.

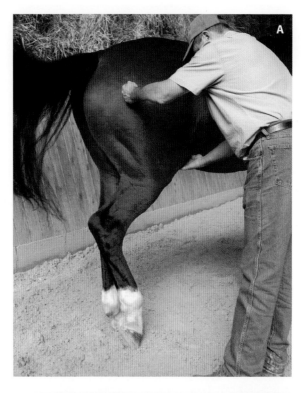

7.20 A & B Be careful when first touching the Stifle Point. The horse can be sore or sensitive in this area (A). Place your hand lower, near the hock, and gently slide up to the Stifle Point (B).

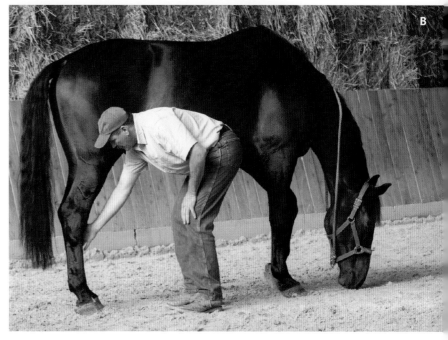

6. The Pubic Symphysis (PS) Point.

The *pubic symphysis* is where the pelvis joins together behind—under the tail. Some hamstring muscles attach here, as well as some fascial attachments that are related to the abdomen, which may have something to do with the breathing response the horse often gives at this point.

There is a horizontal "ridge" or firm band about 3 to 4 inches below the anus, running between the two seat bones, or *ischial tuberosities.* The *Pubic Symphysis Point* is in the middle of this ridge or band (see fig. 7.6, p. 107).

Use this point when the horse is tight in the hamstrings and sacrum, cow-hocked, or appears to be "clamped in" behind. Horses that are tight in the hind part of the groin, as opposed to the stifle area or forward part of the groin, will respond well to this point.

How Release Points are Discovered

I discovered this point—or rather, the horse showed me this point—while working on a horse that was extremely clamped down and tight in the sacrum, hamstrings, and groin muscles behind (as opposed to the forward groin in the stifle area). He was standing excessively cow-hocked, and had trouble releasing his hind leg forward and under as well as back. While searching for areas of tightness, or anywhere that might loosen up the pelvic area, and watching the horse's responses, I happened to get a slight blink at this point. I waited on the spot, and after a short period of time the horse started to breathe heavily, and then started yawning and rolling his eyes repeatedly—classic large release signs. He relaxed behind and started to shift leg to leg. The hamstrings softened, I could manipulate the leg more freely. In short, it worked.

In any case, it works on horses tight in this area, and is worth spending some time searching here for a response.

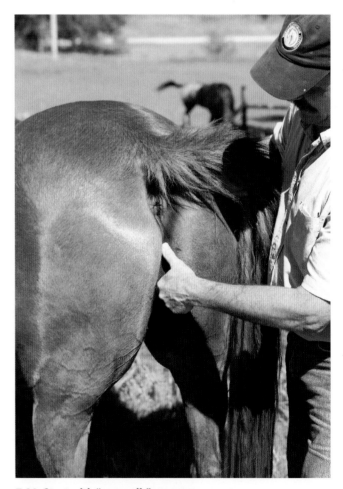

7.21 Start with "egg-yolk" pressure.

Tips

- You may be able to start with a little more pressure such as *egg yolk* to soft *grape* pressure here (fig. 7.21).

- Look for a change in breathing, especially a deeper breathing. This means it is working.

- Once the horse begins to relax into this, you may feel the ridge soften. Gently increase to as much as *grape* pressure. Follow the blinks. Let the horse's responses be your guide. If in doubt, *less is more* (your mantra!).

- On mares, this point will be behind the vulva. You may find the point by going below or to the side of the vulva, then moving toward the midline of the pubic symphysis.

Final Suggestions for Working on Release Points

1. It's important to remember that while working *From the Top* you are *not massaging or pushing* on these points. You are simply sending signals to the horse's nervous system to let go of tension in the hind end.

2. You will see while experimenting with these points that certain ones work better on certain

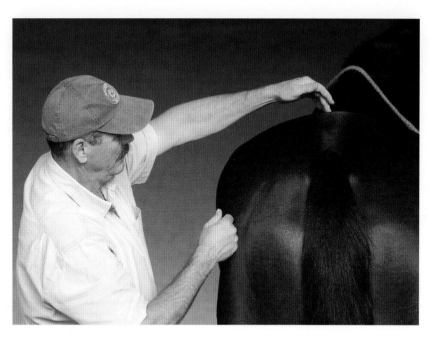

7.22 You can use two points at the same time.

horses and in different orders and combinations, so it isn't necessary to do them in any particular order. However, as I said earlier, I have found it works well to start with one of the *Under-the-Tail Points* first. While you don't have to do both of these points one after the other, be sure that you get both sides done at some time during the process.

3. As stated before, you can apply light touch with *soft* hand, or light touch with a *hard* hand. The horse's nervous system prefers *soft,* and you will get better results with a *soft* hand. So, consciously keep your hand soft while using these points.

4. Every so often, while you are waiting on a spot for some sign of a release, consciously soften your hand while paying very close attention to the horse's eyes. As you soften your hand, you will see a slight softening in the eyes. *As you soften, the* *horse softens.* When the horse softens, he begins to relax and release tension. Simple as that!

5. You may use two points at a time, as long as you are able to read what is going on with the horse's responses with one or both points (fig. 7.22).

6. Think of releasing tension as peeling the layers of an onion (Tears don't usually accompany this process, but don't be surprised if after a large, unexpected release of tension you don't dampen up a bit.) The horse may not release all of the tension in an area in one pass or one session. You may have to peel multiple layers over many sessions, especially if what's creating the tension to start with is not taken care of.

7. If *the horse appears not to be releasing, step back and take a break.* Some horses just don't want to show you the release, or any other sign of submission or giving in. The tension they're holding is often deep stuff that their survival instincts don't want them to reveal.

8. If you have started by focusing on the *Under-the-Tail Point* and the horse hasn't dropped a hip within a minute or two, then you might try the very sensitive *Pelvic Point* to encourage the drop. Or, you may ask the horse to shift his weight to one leg with light pressure on the *hip joint* to start the process.

9. Remember the two principles of the horse's survival instincts:

a) Flee or brace. By staying light you stay under the bracing response. You bring his attention to the tension in a way that allows him to drop his guard. By yielding even slightly to the horse's bracing instinct, you give him nothing to brace against, and he relaxes and releases tension.

b) Herd instinct and body language. The horse's survival depends on body language in the herd. He uses body language to disguise pain, discomfort, and lameness. By observing subtle changes in his behavior or body language, you can find these areas of discomfort and use the correct level of touch to release them (see p. 6 for touch pressures).

> **REMEMBER:**
> If you stay long enough and light enough anywhere the horse tells you he has tension, the horse's nervous system will release that tension.

Technique 2:
WORKING THE HIND END—
FROM THE BOTTOM

GOAL: To use *positioning* and *movement* of the hind limbs to further release tension in the muscles and structure of the hind end.

RESULT: By placing the hind limbs in certain *positions* you allow for a further release of tension beyond the normal point of restriction. *Movement* through certain ranges of motion in a relaxed state further releases tension in major muscles and connective tissue of the sacroiliac, the hind limbs, and the pelvic structure to which they are attached. This uses the *principle of moving a joint or junction through a range of motion in a relaxed state to release tension in the joint or junction.*

HOW IT WORKS

Working the Hind End—From the Bottom involves handling the hind legs in a way similar to the *Scapula Release Techniques* in the front end (p. 62). When you ask the horse to release or "drop" the hind leg in a relaxed state you are also releasing tension in the *Sacroiliac Joint,* similar to the release you get in the *Neck-Shoulder-Withers Junction* with the *Scapula Releases* in the front end. As with the Scapula Releases, there are two parts to this Technique:

Part A: *Releasing the Hind Leg—Down and Forward (p. 126).*

Part B: *Releasing the Hind Leg—Down and Back (p. 137).*

Keep in mind that you are working not only with the limbs, but with the whole structure of the hind end: the lumbar area, pelvis, sacroiliac joint, gluteals, hamstrings, groin, and deeper muscles, such as the psoas, that can neither be seen nor felt from the outside.

Working the Hind End—From the Bottom also helps the horse to release tension in the muscles and structures of the legs such as *stifles, quadriceps, femoral biceps, hamstrings,* and *hocks* by moving these joints and junctions through their range of movement in a relaxed state. The positions used in this Technique also begin to release tension in the lumbar area—even before you begin working on the horse's back.

KEYS TO SUCCESS

- Use your sense of feel and yielding to resistance.

- Feel for the release.

- Pay attention to the horse's responses.

Now, I start Part A: Releasing the Hind Leg—*Down and Forward.*

TECHNIQUE 2: WORKING THE HIND END—*FROM THE BOTTOM*
Part A. Releasing the Hind Leg—Down and Forward

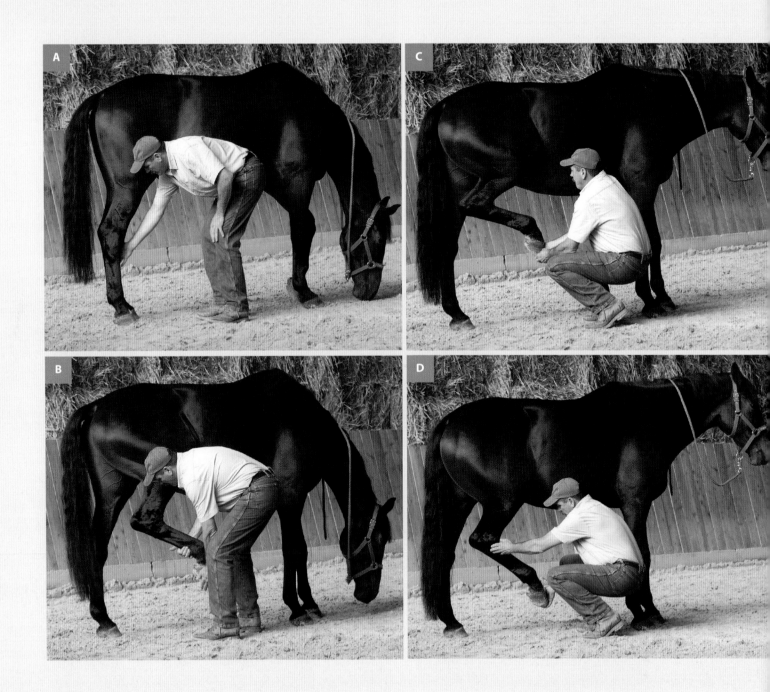

QUICK OVERVIEW: Step-by-Step

TECHNIQUE 2: WORKING THE HIND END—*FROM THE BOTTOM*
Part A. Releasing the Hind Leg—Down and Forward

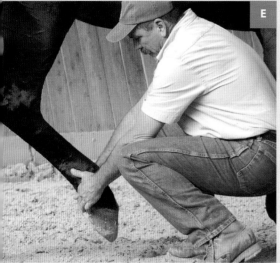

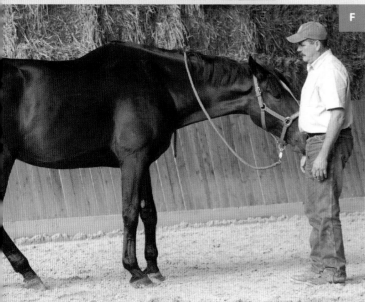

(Starting on Right Side)

Step 1. Stand at the horse's flank, facing toward the rear (A).

Step 2. Ask for the horse's hind leg.

Step 3. As the horse picks the foot up, slide the fingers of one hand under the toe (B).

Step 4. Rest the foot in the "farrier position" giving the horse a chance to relax the leg. Position yourself to protect your back (C).

Step 5. Lower the foot forward to ground, supporting the weight of the leg as you go (D).

Step 6. Slip one hand under the fetlock as the foot nears the ground so that you can gently let go of the toe before the foot touches the ground (E). Keep one hand on the leg to encourage the horse to rest the leg there.

Step 7. Step back and watch for responses (F). If the horse remains in this position, allow him to process the release.

Note: *The absolute best way to practice these Hind Leg Techniques is to enlist the aid of a pony, or if that fails, perhaps a small horse. This way you can get comfortable and familiar with body and leg positions, and movements, without the added struggle of hoisting around 100 pounds of the horse's leg. I can say from experience that the typical hard-nosed horse person will take up this challenge by grabbing the first half-tame Trakehner/ Mustang stallion within reach and start pulling on his legs. But my advice is still to find a pony, pretend nobody else is watching, take it easy on yourself, and learn how to perform the moves without your back going out. Enough said on this one!*

Take Care of Your Back

The horse's hind legs can be heavy so find a body position that allows you to work safely and effectively. Be aware of how you are going to bend, stoop, and stand so you don't harm yourself. You can even get down on your knee—if comfortable, but make sure, though, that the horse has room to move away from you if he gets a sudden urge to relocate!

When you are more comfortable stooping or standing, rest your elbows on your knees to support your back (figs. 7.24 A & B). You will eventually develop your own positions and style of comfortably handling the hind legs.

Safety Note: The hind end can be "loaded." When first asking a horse to lift a hind leg, the safest place to stand is a little farther forward near the flank of the horse, facing toward the hind end. Then, if the horse unexpectedly kicks out, you are not in the immediate firing range. By the time you get to working with the hind end, you should be comfortable with the horse and he should be comfortable with you. Still, be aware that the horse may have some sensitive or sore muscles.

7.24 A & B If standing, brace your elbow on your knee to support your back (A). You can support the leg while on one knee (B).

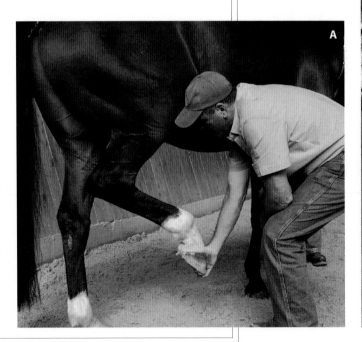

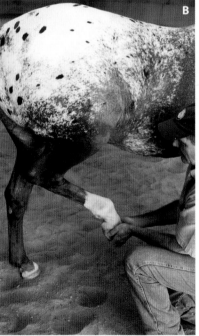

Part A. Releasing the Hind Leg Down and Forward in More Detail

1. Position the horse.

Position him in the stall in a place that is safe for both you and him. The best place is in the center of the stall where he has room to move away from you. The worst place is with him against the wall and you on the open side, meaning his only escape route is through you. Make sure that he is not backed against or too close to the wall with his hind end.

Be sure that the horse is standing somewhat square. Whenever you pick up any one of his legs you want to be sure he has his balance and won't have to step or fall forward or back.

2. Position yourself.

Stand next to the horse's hind end as if to pick up his hoof for cleaning, facing toward the rear. If the horse is unfamiliar to you, stand a little more toward his belly.

3. Pick up the foot.

When asking the horse to pick up the leg, shift your weight gently toward him, place your hand on his pastern or cannon bone and ask by gently squeezing. When he begins to shift his weight off the foot or picks the foot up, soften your grip to let him know that's what you want. Ask, release, ask, release, until he lifts the foot. Pretty soon he'll be lifting his own leg every time you put your hand there.

As he picks it up slide your hand under the pastern, or if you are comfortable, under the toe. Wait for him to relax into your hand, then take a short step backward (toward the horse's head) and bring the foot forward just a little bit.

Remember to find a comfortable position for you that makes it easy on your back. Close to the horse's body is better. Rest your elbows on your knees to support your back as you give the horse a minute to relax the leg, pelvis, and lower back.

4. Handle the feet and legs in a way that makes it easy for the horse to yield to you.

Don't grab and pull: Once the foot is off the ground, the best way to get kicked is to grab the cannon bone and pull when the horse pulls away. Slide your hand from the cannon bone to under the pastern, or slip your fingers under the front of the toe and bring the foot forward. Use the same yielding sense of "feel" that you have developed with previous Techniques such as *Lateral Cervical Flexion* (p. 33). Be ready to support the weight when the horse relaxes the leg.

5. Support the leg once it is off the ground.

After the horse has lifted the leg, you must support the weight of the leg: If you are holding by the toe, the ideal position and distance is about where the foot would be if it were on a hoof stand while being shod. This is why I refer to this position of the leg as the "farrier position." Not only is this the most comfortable position for the horse, but if the horse steps down, you will have time to let go of the toe.

6. Consciously feel for signs of relaxation in the horse's leg and hind end.

Signs of relaxation will be when the leg gets heavier, or when the stifle starts to relax and fall out to the side. Once you feel him start to get heavy in your hand, gently and slowly guide the leg down and forward, and a little toward the midline of the horse, under the belly.

Note: *If you get tired while waiting for the horse to relax through a certain point, you can set the foot down normally, stand up and stretch, then start up where you left off. This is the case with any of these Techniques: You can let go, and then pick up again at any point in the process. You may notice that each time you do this, the hind limb will be more relaxed (and heavier, sorry), and that it will be easier for him to do the release.*

7. Lower the foot to the ground.

It's important to support the weight of the leg as

you lower it to the ground. As the foot gets closer to the ground, slide one hand behind the pastern and lift under the ankle as you remove the fingers of the other hand from under the toe. Remember to *lift* under the pastern *before* you let go under the toe. This way the horse will stay relaxed in your hand. If you let go of the toe before supporting the ankle, the horse will lift his leg up.

Best Trick for Handling Feet and Legs

If you've ever watched a good farrier (they're out there!) pick up a difficult horse's foot, you're likely to see him hold the foot by the toe until the horse stops struggling. Holding the toe not only makes it easier to hold the foot but also makes it much easier for the horse to relax the foot and leg into your hand.

Note: When holding the toe it's important to be aware of when it's time to let go. One of those times is when the horse gets so agitated that it becomes dangerous for you (or him) to continue. Once you get used to yielding to resistance while holding the toe, it will be possible for you to relax many a distraught horse.

I don't want to make a big deal of this, but when it's done properly, handling the foot by the toe is the best way to work with most horses. The main point I want to get across is: When you handle the horse by the toe, the absolute best time to let go is before the foot is planted firmly on the ground.

8. Pick a spot on the ground.

You need a general landing spot for the foot. Look for a spot where the horse may comfortably be able to rest the leg. Feel for this spot as you lower the leg. You are looking for a little more forward and under than he would normally rest it on his own.

Note: Don't ask him to bring the leg too far forward the first time. It's better to give him a more comfortable position that he can relax in longer, than a more stretched position that he has trouble relaxing into. Remember, you're peeling layers off of the onion, one by one.

9. Rest the foot.

Once the foot is resting on the ground keep your hand on the foot or on the leg to encourage the horse to stay in this position. Most horses will pick the foot back up when you take your hand off the foot or leg.

You eventually want the foot to rest on the ground in a position as far forward and under as the horse can comfortably rest it, while keeping weight on the opposite leg (fig. 7.25). The longer he is able to relax in this position the more he will release. This is what I call "Horse Yoga" for the hind end. Leave the horse in this position until he comes out of it. He will go into a seemingly "drugged" state. I suspect the "drugs" are endorphins! If you have the time, allow him to stay in this position for as long as he likes. Apart from a good rest, he will have a very relaxed hind end.

Notice the following:

- How much lower the pelvis drops the longer the horse stays in this position.

- How much lower it is each time he does it.

- How much of a relaxed "twist" there is in the lumbar spine with the hip dropped.

10. Take a step back.

See what the horse has to say. If your horse leaves the leg in this position then let him process through the release until he steps out of it on his own. Sometimes the horse will show you *visible release responses* right away, sometimes he will *stand and process* (see below) then show releases after he is done, or *show no responses* at all. This depends on the horse: the amount of tension he may have had, how much he released, and whether he's comfortable showing it to you or not.

Note on Processing: *Sometimes the horse will stay in this leg forward-and-under position for any-where from a few seconds, to even a few minutes, especially when the leg is on or crossed over the midline. This is not only because it feels good after having released tension, but because his nervous system may be processing the release. It will appear that he is either staring off in the distance, or that he is half asleep with his head down. The difference will be that his lips will twitch, his eyes will blink or widen and then go to half-mast, and every once in a while his body will kind of jerk as if he's got a little electric shock.*

Don't panic, stay calm! This is good.

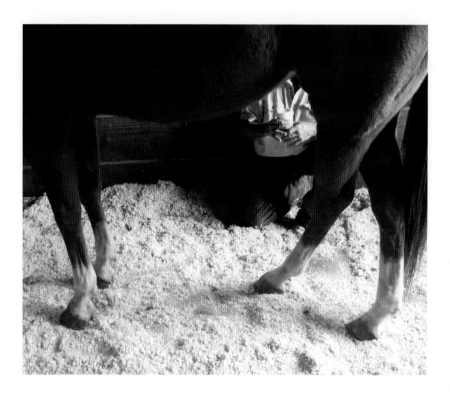

7.25 This horse is resting with the leg down and forward across the midline.

What Ifs?

- ***What if the horse pulls the leg up during the process?***

At some point while lowering the leg, the horse will likely pull his leg up. This is normal. When it happens, don't pull back on the leg, but *yield* to the horse (fig. 7.26 A). Keep your hand on the toe or ankle, and go up with the leg. Just keep him "in the neighborhood" until he relaxes into your hand again (fig. 7.26 B).

As he relaxes into your hand be ready to immediately support the weight of the leg in the "farrier position," then continue lowering the leg while supporting the weight as much as possible.

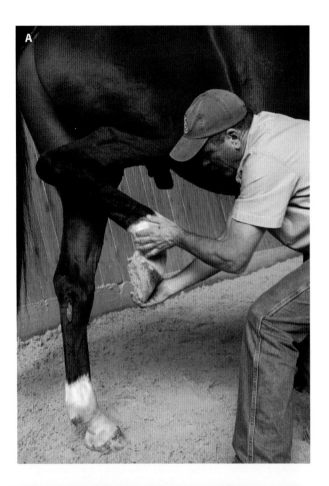

7.26 A & B If the horse pulls the leg up, keep your hands on the leg but don't pull back (A). Just go with the horse, and wait until he rests the leg back in your hand (B).

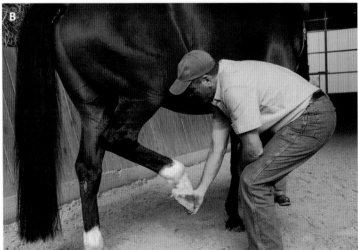

■ *Why is the horse pulling his leg up?*

He is likely relaxing into a point of restriction somewhere in the hind end and the discomfort causes him to pull the leg up.

Each time he pulls up, he is releasing some of the tension or restriction. This may happen multiple times, depending on how much tension or restriction is there. Each time you will feel the leg more relaxed.

■ *What if my horse resists releasing the leg down?*

It is an indication that there is pain or restriction in the hind end, which means you will help him by releasing it. Supporting the leg more—or longer—will make it easier for him to relax it, as described above.

Whenever the horse shows you he is uncomfortable with anything you ask of the hind legs, bring the leg back to the farrier position and wait for him to relax into it. This is the "default" position.

When it's time to relax the leg down, make it easier for him by asking him to set it down just a short distance forward, rather than farther away (figs. 7.27 A & B). Give him a position that he can stay in longer. The more time he can comfortably stay in a position, the better the release.

In some cases, the horse may not be able to reach the ground in this position, in a relaxed state. In this case, support the weight of the foot and leg in your hand. Sometimes you may have to hold it up off of the ground for quite a while. If you are working in shavings you can make a small pile

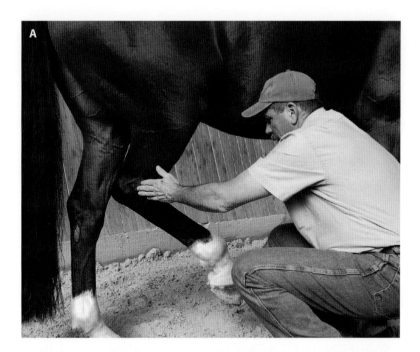

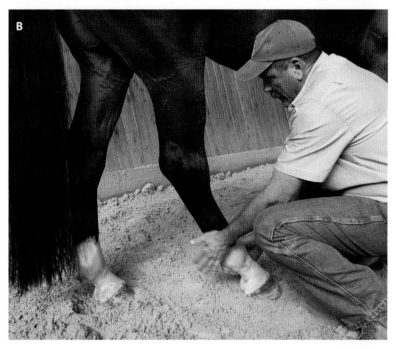

7.27 A & B Make it easier for your horse by asking him to set his foot down just a short distance forward.

A Lesson in How the Horse Releases Tension

E arly on when I started doing this Technique, sometimes a horse would have so much tension up above that he couldn't relax the leg all the way to the ground. I would try to hold the foot up as long as possible but he would push all his weight into my hand, the toe would slip out of my fingers, and the foot would stomp to the ground. The first few times it happened I became pretty discouraged, thinking it wasn't working. But then I started to notice that each time this happened, when I tried again, the leg became more and more relaxed as I let it down, and the horse would be more relaxed in the *sacrolumbar* area each time this happened.

It soon became clear that when I ran into resistance it meant that the horse had relaxed into a point of discomfort or restriction, and that if I held just a second longer before yielding that he would release some of that tension. When I came back to try again, the horse would be softer and able to more comfortably move through what I was asking. This was often followed by the visible release responses.

The moral is: Sometimes discomfort and resistance go along with the release.

Also, sometimes you don't think you're getting the work done, but, in fact, you are.

of them so that the horse can rest his toe on that. The goal is to have the foot and leg *relaxed* in this position.

Keep in mind that each time he pulls his leg up, he is releasing some tension or restriction. This may happen multiple times, depending on how much tension or restriction is there. Each time you will feel the horse more comfortable relaxing the leg down again and able to relax it a little farther forward.

■ *What if my horse quickly puts the foot down, or puts all of his weight on it without relaxing it?*

This will happen. Sometimes the horse just thinks that's what you're asking him to do. Slow the process down, as if you were asking him to gently set the foot down. If you can keep his weight on the opposite leg just a little bit as he sets this one down, it will give him a chance to release a little bit each time, and it will get progressively better. All you are looking for at each step of the way is an *improvement*. Don't try to get the "full Monty" all in one go.

If he needs to put his foot down before you are ready, try to guide it down to a spot close in, and let go. Also, be sure that:

1. The horse was standing square when you picked up the leg.

2. You are not asking him to step too far.

3. You are not pulling him a little off balance. When you ask the horse to position the leg you need to allow him to keep his balance on the other three legs.

Usually when the horse is uncomfortable, it means he is just at the moment where he is ready to release that tension. It's your job to support him through that point.

■ *What if my horse does not want to keep the leg in this position once the foot is down. Does this mean he is not releasing or processing?*

The horse will process after a release no matter what, even after returning to a normal standing position. If the horse is able to stay in the position longer, he will release longer, but sometimes you have to take it in little chunks.

One reason the horse may not stay in the release position longer is that he may still not be able to relax comfortably in that position as there is still tension to release. There may still be layers of the onion to peel.

Kicking as a Form of Communication

In my experience, most of the time when the horse kicks out, he isn't trying to kick you. If he really means to kick you, he can and will, no matter how fast you react. Kicking is kicking. But when the horse kicks at you or threatens you, he is letting you know he dislikes whatever it is you're doing. It's a form of communication. You have to decide how you're going to respond to this. Remember, your safety comes first.

Another is that he may not be comfortable with a human doing this with him and he may be guarded or defensive. All horses are different.

■ *What if the horse kicks out or threatens to kick?*

First of all remember: Your safety comes first! If you are concerned about it, take a step back. Below are some guidelines that might help you interpret the horse's behavior and decide how to handle this scenario:

1. When you first ask the horse to pick up the foot, it's basically the same request as when you want to clean it. In that case, you just deal with it normally. But when you're going to pick it up for this exercise, the horse should be trained to do it safely.

2. If the horse is so sore that he's uncomfortable about you touching him, which may be why you're there in the first place, it may be better to work *From the Top* for a while, or exclusively.

3. If you approach a horse that *really* threatens you, and it's clear that he's serious about keeping you out of range, then *stay out of range!* There's either a serious physical issue or a serious training issue.

4. When the horse becomes uncomfortable while you are lowering the leg and wants to kick, it is safer to be holding the toe as described earlier, and for the same reasons (see p. 130). You are safer when control the foot.

5. If the horse becomes too uncomfortable then let the foot down, give the horse (and yourself) a breather, then ask again.

Response—or Perhaps Not?

Don't be discouraged if you feel like you're not getting the responses you're expecting. If you do these Techniques with the horse in as relaxed a state as he can be in, he will release some tension and his body will process it, even if he doesn't show it to you.

A lot of these things will become more apparent to you after you have done these exercises a few times. If you are doing these Techniques even close to as described in this book, the horse will release.

■ *How many times should I repeat this exercise within one session?*

If the horse can easily do what you're asking and relaxes the leg down in one try, then once is enough! If the horse has difficulty with it, you may want to do it a few times, feeling for *improvement* each time. In this case, try to go slower the second time, giving the horse a chance to *relax into the release*.

Also, it's important to break it up a little by going from one side to the other, or doing another Technique then coming back to this one. If you repeat a Technique more than two or three times in a row, the horse will quickly learn to either go through the exercise without relaxing, or to simply evade doing it altogether.

A Horse Can Work with Stringhalt

Stringhalt ("shivers"): The last thing to mention is the possibility of stringhalt in the hind limb or limbs. This is something the horse has no control over. It can range from severe to mild. With mild stringhalt, the horse can eventually relax the leg into your hand. In severe cases, the horse can't relax the leg at all when it's picked up, and will continue to spasm until you let go of the leg. This condition is a neurological proprioception issue:, meaning that the horse can raise the leg on his own, but his nervous system loses awareness of the leg's position when it is picked up by someone else.

I worked on a show hunter on a regular basis that had stringhalt so severe he needed to be sedated in order to have either hind foot picked up, yet he could pick up his feet on his own and was a very successful A level competitor. I was also able to successfully keep this horse free and loose in the hind end using the *Working From the Top* Techniques in this book. Kept us both happy.

In most cases you won't release *all* of the tension in one session, especially if the horse is in work, or whatever is causing the tension is still there. But you will make an improvement each time. Each time you repeat a Technique, or a session with the horse, look (or feel) for the improvement.

■ *What if the horse has trouble relaxing in the leg forward position?*

As with the preceding question, often, once isn't enough. Also, every horse is different. They all have different issues, levels of tension, and body types, and react differently to your attempts to help them release tension. Some hold on to tension more than others, some let go more readily. You may notice this reflected in their personality. As long as you make an improvement each time, you are making progress.

Note: *Be aware of possible pain or injury in the horse. If he consistently or absolutely refuses to either hold up the leg or relax it to the ground keep in mind the possibility of pain or injury. A sore or injured hock, leg, stifle or soreness farther up in the lumbar and pelvic area may make it difficult for the horse to hold the leg up. In addition, a sore hock, leg or stifle on the opposite side may make it difficult for the horse to stand on that leg when asked to lift the leg you are working with.*

Next I'll discuss *Technique 2, Part B: Releasing the Hind Leg—Down and Back.*

QUICK OVERVIEW: Step-by-Step

TECHNIQUE 2: WORKING THE HIND END—*FROM THE BOTTOM*
Part B: Releasing the Hind Leg—Down and Back

Step 1. Stand next to the horse's hip, facing the rear (A).

Step 2. Ask for the horse's foot, as if going to clean the hoof (B).

Step 3. Hold the foot by the pastern, with the ankle bent. Keep your hand soft.

Step 4. As the horse relaxes the leg, guide it down and back to rest with the toe on the ground (C).

Step 5. When the leg has relaxed, wiggle it gently to encourage more relaxation, and slide the toe farther back (D).

Step 6. Keep your hand on the leg to encourage the horse to rest in this position.

Step 7. Step back and see what the horse has to say (E).

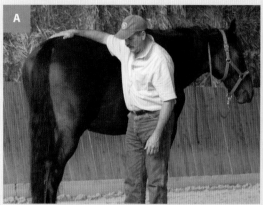

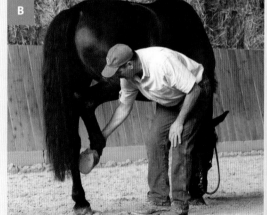

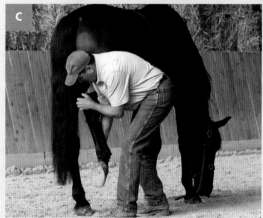

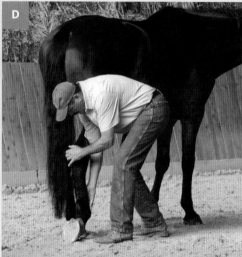

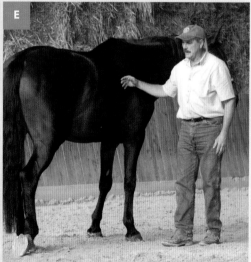

Part B. Releasing the Hind Leg Down and Back in More Detail

1. Position the horse.

Use the center of the stall. If he has the urge to go somewhere quickly, it's better that he has enough room to move *away* from you. Also, make sure he is standing reasonably square so that he can remain relaxed and easily keep his balance. Do not position his hind end close to the wall. He may kick out and you or your hand could possibly get between his foot and the wall.

2. Position yourself.

Stand next to the horse's hind end as if to pick up his hoof for cleaning, facing toward the rear. Stay out of his "kick zone." If he wants to kick, he will, but if he kicks out as a reaction to something else, you don't want to be in the way.

3. Ask the horse to pick up the foot.

"Ask" is the key word here. When you have it in mind that you are simply asking for the foot to clean the hoof, most horses will comply without a fuss. When he has picked the foot up, wait for him to relax the leg. Don't grab it.

4. Relax the leg down and back.

With your hand in front of the pastern, guide the leg back so that his pastern is bent and he is resting his toe a few inches behind the other foot. The first time you ask, it is better to rest the toe only a few inches farther back than the other foot. After the horse has really relaxed in this position, slide the toe back another inch or so. This way, you can

gradually extend the range of *relaxed* position and movement.

The longer he is able to relax in this position the more he will release so it's better to give him a more comfortable position that he can relax into longer, rather than a more stretched position that he has trouble relaxing into.

5. Keep your hand on the foot or on the leg.

It encourages the horse to stay in this position longer. Most horses will pick the foot back up when you take your hand off.

6. Consciously feel and look for signs of relaxation.

Some signs of relaxation in the horse's leg and pelvis will be when the pastern lowers closer to the ground, the hip or pelvis relaxes and drops lower, the breathing changes, the eyes close and the head drops.

As with *Releasing the Leg—Down and Forward,* when the horse has tension or discomfort in either the hock, stifle, muscles of the hamstrings, gluteals, pelvis or even lower back, he may pull the leg back up. When this happens don't pull on the leg, but yield to the horse. Keep your hand on the foot or pastern and go up with the leg. Just "keep him in the neighborhood" until he relaxes, then guide the leg down again to a more comfortable position.

In some cases, the horse may not be able to comfortably reach the ground in this position. In this case, with the foot back, hold the foot under the front of the pastern with the ankle bent, and support the weight of the foot and leg in your hand. Sometimes you may have to hold it up off the ground for quite a while. As mentioned earlier, when you are working in shavings you can make a small pile so that the horse may rest his toe on it. The goal is to have the foot and leg *relaxed* in this position.

Note: *Remember that each time he pulls up, he is releasing some tension or restriction. This may happen multiple times, depending on how much tension or restriction is there. Each time you will feel the horse more comfortable relaxing the leg back again, and able to relax it back a little further.*

Notice the following:

■ How much lower the pelvis drops the longer the horse stays in this position.

■ How much lower it is each time he does it.

■ How much of a relaxed "twist" there is in the lumbar area with the hip dropped.

   Any movement—no matter how slow or subtle—of a joint or junction, including the vertebrae of the lower back, through a range of motion in a relaxed state, releases tension in that joint or junction. This is what is happening when the horse relaxes the hip into this dropped position (fig. 7.29).

   This relaxed leg-back position has a powerful effect on the lower back, as it relaxes tension in the largest *driving muscle* in the horse—the middle gluteal (gluteus medius)—that attaches at the front end in the lumbar region and at the back end on the greater trochanter of the femur at the hip joint (see fig. 7.4, p. 106) This means that

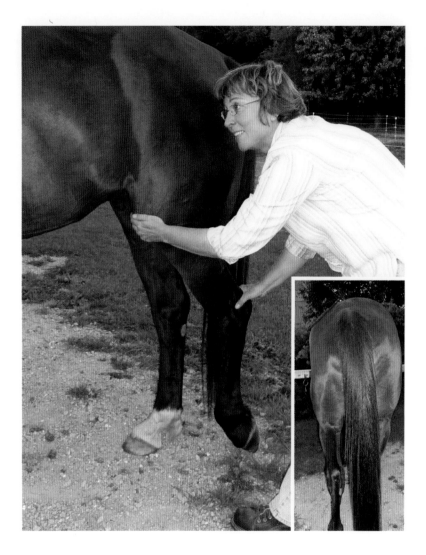

the tension on the lower back is relaxed. Relaxing this area also relaxes the psoas muscles, which are underneath the lumbar spine (see figs. 7.6 and 7.9, pp. 107 and 110).

7. Things you can do while the leg is resting back.

Once the leg has relaxed in this position you can *gently* massage the softened hamstring muscles,

7.29 The horse drops the hip in the "leg back" position and releases tension in the lumbar area.

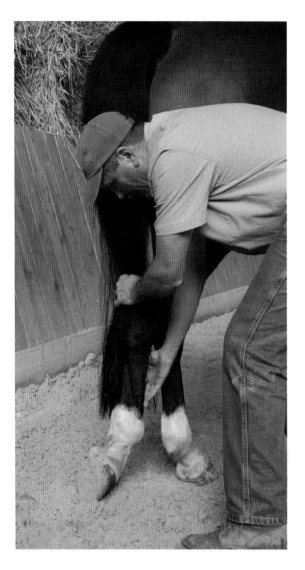

7.30 When the horse has relaxed on the toe in this position, you may slide the toe a little farther back.

and the muscles of the lumbar area. Wiggle the leg gently to encourage the horse to relax it even more. If the horse tenses, stop wiggling or wiggle softer.

Once the horse has relaxed the pastern down in this position, you may slide the toe a little farther back (fig. 7.30). Wait for him to relax and drop the hip even more while in this position. If he

picks the foot up, don't struggle with him, just gently ask again.

8. Step back and see what he has to say.

This is a very powerful position for horses with soreness or restriction in the lower back. You may be surprised how much tension the horse will release here. If he stays in this position on his own for a while—good!

Safety Note for the Horse: Be careful, as you bring the leg back, not to allow the horse to step back onto his pastern! If he starts to shift his weight back, release his foot so that he can step down on the sole of the foot without buckling onto his pastern. Allow the horse to keep his balance on the other three legs: If you pull his leg back, or bring the leg back too far and don't let go, he could hyperextend the leg and/or lock his stifle.

Don't pull, be careful, and be aware of the horse's balance! And remember: Before you begin, make sure he is standing reasonably square before picking up his leg.

Safety Note for You: Remember to position the horse so that his hind end is away from the wall when doing this Technique. If he were to kick out with your hand on his foot near the wall, you may get your hand hurt. Stand facing toward the tail and as far forward of the leg as you comfortably can while doing these releases. This minimizes the risk of getting hit with a wayward foot.

Important: Whether you are nervous handling the legs or not, you have to have confidence in what you are doing or the horse will notice, and you'll both be nervous. You must be confident in order to be safe.

What Ifs?

■ *What if he doesn't want to rest the leg down and back, or picks it up as I set it back?*

If the horse is uncomfortable releasing the leg back, it's an indication that there may be pain or restriction in the hind end; either the hip-gluteal or often, the sacrolumbar area. It is also a sign that you will help him by releasing it.

Start by asking him to pick up the foot for cleaning. Sometimes it helps to actually clean it a little, as (we hope) he is used to that.

From there, if he starts to relax the leg, slowly guide it down with the ankle bent and in the direction you want to go until the toe touches the ground. If he lifts up before then, keep your hand softly on the front of his ankle and go with him, keeping him "in the neighborhood" waiting until he relaxes it down again. Then, guide the toe back down (figs. 7.31 A–C). You may have to support the weight of the leg by the front of the pastern until he is ready to relax through that point of restriction.

By the way, if you are asking the horse to bring the leg too far back, and he has sore stifles, then it may be uncomfortable for him to relax through the discomfort into this position.

Note: *It may help to support the leg, or use a little pressure and encouragement to ask him to bring it down and back. However, DON'T get into a tug of war with the hind leg in this position! The human challenger very rarely comes out on top in this particular competition.*

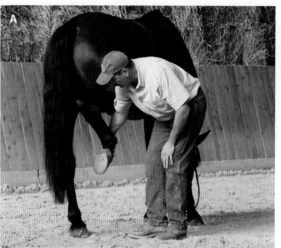
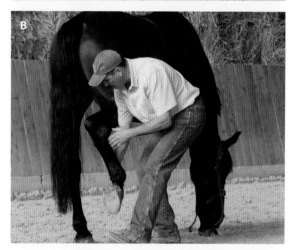
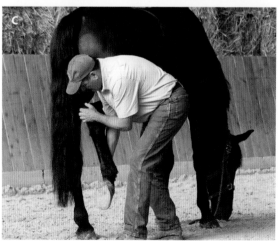

7.31 A–C If he pulls the leg up, don't pull back (A). Keep your hand softly on the leg and go with him, keeping him "in the neighborhood" (B). When he relaxes it down again, guide the toe back where you want it (C).

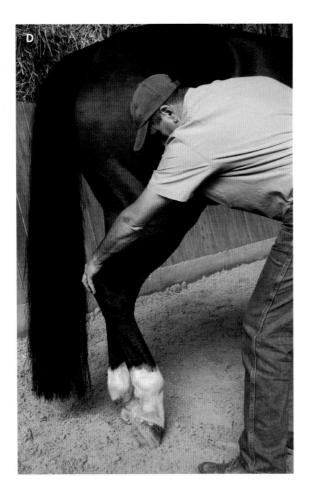

7.31 D It may make it easier for both you and the horse if you first ask him to set the foot down right next to the other foot.

You *may* be asking him to bring the foot farther back than he is comfortable doing. It may make it easier for both you and the horse if, the first time, you ask him to set the foot down right next to the other foot (fig. 7.31 D). Once he is resting in that position you can gently slide his toe back an inch or two when he isn't looking.

■ *Can I keep sliding the toe farther back?*

Yes. Once he is relaxed with his toe resting down and back you can slide the toe farther back to extend the leg farther out. This extension of the leg releases tension in the muscles of the leg and back, and is good for the stifles and hocks as long as the leg stays relaxed.

Safety Note: Remember to be careful not to pull the horse off balance with his foot in your hand. If he steps back and you are holding his leg he may hyperextend or buckle onto his pastern. Should this happen, let go of the leg.

■ *What if his foot crosses over in back?*

This is okay. Guide the foot down wherever it is most comfortable for the horse. Due to conformational factors or muscle-tightness issues, different horses are comfortable resting their feet in different positions. The best place to start with any Technique is where the horse is most comfortable, and then to help the horse gradually move out from there in a relaxed state.

A Final Note on the Hind Leg Releases

You'll be surprised how much improvement you can achieve in only a few sessions with these Techniques. You may notice when coming back to perform the Techniques later that the leg feels easier to manipulate than when you first started out.

The movements you get with the Hind Leg Releases can be much more subtle than the movements you get from the front end. However, the releases and the responses, such as yawning, eye-rolling, snorting, head-shaking, can be just as powerful.

CHAPTER 8

Working Toward the Middle—The Horse's Back

Technique 1:
LATERAL ROCKING

Before You Begin

GOAL: To gently rock the horse's spinal column side to side, from head to tail, in a relaxed state. This creates movement in the soft tissue between the individual vertebrae of the spinal column.

RESULT: Increased comfort and suppleness in the spine and more efficient use of the hind limbs forward through the body. Movement of these joints through even a tiny range of motion in a relaxed state releases tension in the muscles surrounding these joints.

WHERE YOU WORK—ANATOMY

Spinal Column

The horse's spinal column is a chain of interconnected vertebrae which are anatomically divided into four sections, not including the tail.

The cervical spine: You learned how to release tension in the seven vertebrae of the neck in the first chapter (p. 2).

The thoracic spine: This is made up of the vertebrae of the horse's trunk and rib cage and includes the withers and mid back. Each thoracic vertebra has a corresponding rib. There are normally 18 thoracic vertebrae and ribs.

The lumbar spine: These are the vertebrae of the lower back. They begin where the rib cage ends, approximately where the back of the saddle

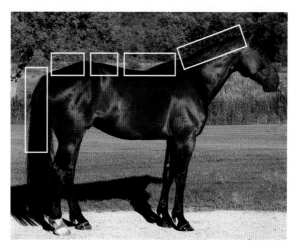

8.1 A **The five sections of the horse's spine.**

rests. They do not have ribs, but have large flat *transverse processes* ("wings"), which provide anchor points for powerful back muscles. There are normally six lumbar vertebrae.

The sacrum: This comprises the last five vertebrae of the spinal column fused together into one bone.

The tail: And bringing up the rear, there are 18 or so *caudal vertebrae.*

With this Technique, especially, it helps to have a good mental picture of the anatomy. It helps to give you a picture of where you place your hands, as well as what is going on up the line with the pelvis, spine, and ribs as you rock the horse.

WHERE YOU WILL PUT YOUR HANDS

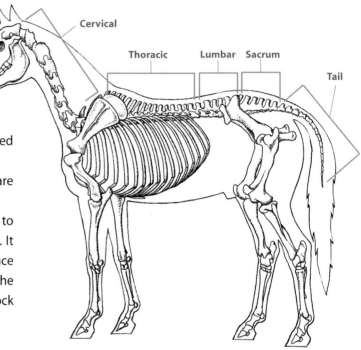

8.1 B The spinal column.

Sacrum

The sacrum is one of the "handles" you use to create waves of motion that travel through the length of the horse's body. Place your hand on the sacrum, where the tail joins it—as high up as possible to allow you to get a solid grip. Get a good feel for where the most solid hand-hold is. This is where you will initiate the movement. This hand will be the "rocking hand."

Pelvis

Feel for the widest point of the pelvis—the hip bone *(tuber coxae).* This solid spot is where you will place your second hand to assist, or augment the movement initiated by the "rocking hand." This hand will be the "helping hand."

Ribs

Next, slide your "helping hand" forward toward the flank. Locate the last rib, then feel each rib as you move your hand forward until you reach the ribs just behind the scapula and withers. Each rib connects with a vertebra. This is where you ask for more movement once you have the horse relaxed. Visualize one rib attached to each vertebra, all joined through cartilage and ultimately connected to the sacrum. The focus of this Technique is is on the 18 thoracic and six lumbar vertebrae that comprise the horse's back (fig. 8.2).

Vertebrae

And finally, to get a feel for how the vertebrae fit together, run your fingers down the center of the back, feeling the *dorsal spinous process* of each individual vertebra. Begin at the withers, down the back, over the lumbar vertebrae, over the sacroiliac joint and over the sacrum to the tail.

Muscles

Some of the muscles (positively) affected by this Technique are:

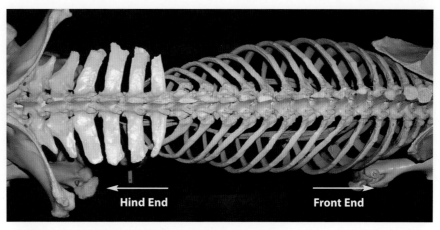

8.2 Thoracic vertebrae (with ribs) and lumbar vertebrae (with "wings") that make up the horse's back.

1. The *multifidi* muscles that intertwine the vertebrae of the spine.
2. The *longissimus dorsi* muscles that go down each side of the back from the pelvis, attaching to the lower neck, and on to the upper neck and poll (fig. 7.9, p. 110).
3. The *iliocostal* muscles (iliocostis) that run from the lumbar spine to the lower neck, and support the *longissimus dorsi*.
4. The *psoas* muscle group that supports the lower back (see fig. 8.9, p. 152).

RELEASING TENSION: THE EFFECTS

Back pain and tension can be exacerbated by issues such as poor saddle fit; improper riding; stifle, hock, or foot pain; or diseases such as EPM or Lyme—to name a couple.

Tension that develops over time will cause rigidity in the back, affecting movement and putting added stress on other parts of the horse. For example, a lower back that is not functioning fully can transfer stress to structures of the hind limb, such as the stifle.

A lower back (lumbar spine) that is restricted in movement (a very common condition) prevents the horse from utilizing his whole body when pushing forward. This is one area that, when released, will make a noticeable difference in the horse's movement, even when there wasn't a

The Importance of a Supple Poll

"Suppleness of the poll is essential to the suppleness of the back; you can't have one without the other," says Sarah Wyche in *Understanding The Horse's Back*. *Lateral Rocking* is a very effective Technique when combined with releasing tension in the poll. If you have a horse that is suffering from a rigid or sore back be sure to combine the *Lateral Rocking Technique* with work on the poll.

QUICK OVERVIEW: Step-by-Step

TECHNIQUE 1: LATERAL ROCKING

Step 1. Stand on the left side of the horse, next to the hip, face forward at about a 30-degree angle (A).

Step 2. Place your right hand on the sacrum at the base of the horse's tail.

Step 3. Place your left hand gently on the point of the horse's left hip (B).

Step 4. With your right hand gently rock the hind end from side to side. Start with "pushing" motions to sway the horse's spine gently from side to side. Continue rocking until you and the horse have a relaxed rhythm.

Step 5. As you rock, slide your left hand directly forward to the area of the last rib. Use the rib to gently rock the corresponding vertebra (C).

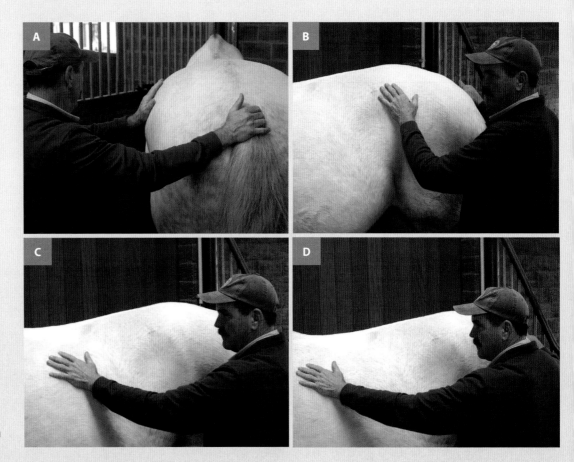

Step 6. Continue moving your left hand forward as you gently rock each rib and vertebra. You can go all the way to behind the withers, if your arms are long enough (D).

noticeable problem before the release. A freely swinging back is important to any functional gait in the horse.

Among other things, a restricted back can result in a short-striding gait. In dressage, for example, the concept of a mental and physical state of relaxation is based on the assumption that the horse is physically able to translate hind-end movement into one fluid motion that travels through the body into the head and allows his back to swing freely. The *Lateral Rocking Technique* encourages this type of movement by releasing tension in the soft tissue surrounding the individual vertebrae. This exercise also simulates natural hind-end movement in the relaxed horse.

You've already learned that moving a joint through its range of motion in a relaxed state releases tension in the muscles and ligaments that surround the joint. *Lateral Rocking* is a gentle, effective way of moving the vertebrae through a small range of motion in a relaxed state, releasing tension and freeing up the back.

Quality Over Quantity

Moving a joint or junction through even a *tiny* range of motion (micro-wiggling) while the horse is relaxed is ten times more effective than moving a joint or junction through a *large* range of motion, in a non-relaxed state.

This is all not to overlook the effect that *Lateral Rocking* will have on breathing. Some of the *Release Points* used in *Working the Hind End—From the Top* have already had a loosening effect on the diaphragm (see p. 111). *Lateral Rocking* will get movement in the ribs and further loosen muscles associated with breathing.

Technique 1 in More Detail

The horse's back is a very rigid structure. Compared to a dog for instance, the horse has relatively little ability to bend laterally in the back and pelvis. Consequently, it can be one of the more difficult areas from which to release deep-seated tension.

Before working on the back, it's best to first loosen up both ends of the horse—as you have done—then work your way toward the middle. Although moving a joint or junction through a range of motion in a relaxed state is now relatively easy for you to apply to a neck or a limb, it will seem a little trickier to do with something as massive as the back.

Not to worry: As there is relatively little movement in the horse's back to begin with, it requires relatively little movement to release tension in it. As with many of these Techniques, it's less a matter of strength or force, but more of feel, rhythm and timing. It may take a few tries to get the rhythm and timing, but be patient; it will happen.

There are two ways to do this *Lateral Rocking Technique*. One is placing your hand at the base of the tail and using the sacrum, as shown in the step-by-step instructions on p. 146. You use the horse's sacrum at the base of the tail as a "handle" in order to send a wave of motion through his body.

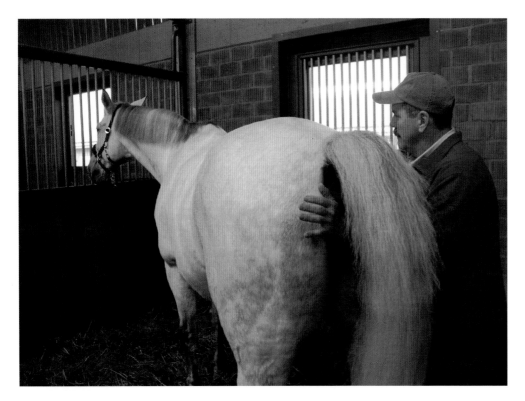

develop just the right rhythm and feel in your own body. A horse that is overly sensitive, keeps walking off, or takes more drastic steps to "get you off of his back," is not the right partner on which to practice developing your rhythm and feel. However, once you are good at this exercise, it is an effective way to release tension in the horse's back.

It is good to perform this Technique on both sides of the back. If there is an indication that one side is either stiffer or more painful than the other, it is better to start on the opposite (meaning easier) side. If there doesn't appear to be a stiffer side, just pick one. I think it's easier to learn with your dominant hand as the rocking hand, so if you are right-handed, start on the left side of the horse, with your right hand on the sacrum at the base of his tail, or on the point of the buttock.

1. Position yourself.

You are going to use a "rocking hand" and a "helping hand."

Stand at the horse's left hip and place your right hand—the rocking hand—on the sacrum. Take a firm grip on the sacrum, as high up the tail as possible so you are not just wagging the tail (an activity for dogs only).

Rest your left, or helping hand, gently on the point of the hip. You will not be using this hand much in the beginning (fig. 8.5).

8.4 Place your "rocking" hand here on the inside of the point of the buttock.

Second, you can also perform this Technique by placing your "rocking hand" on the inside of the point of the buttock *(ischium),* instead of on the base of the tail (fig. 8.4). Standing on the same side of the horse, apply the pushing/rocking force to the bony protuberance of the buttock on the opposite side. On some horses you can get a better purchase with your hand there than you can on the tail.

The key with either is to use the rocking hand to create small "waves" and to do it in a way that keeps the horse relaxed.

Note: *It's best to practice on a horse you are familiar with, and one that is not too uncomfortable when you do the rocking: It takes a little while to*

2. Start with the "rocking hand."

With the rocking hand, begin by asking for very small side-to-side movements until you, and the horse, get the rhythm and you feel him start to soften and relax. Keep your arm slightly bent but firm, so that you can use your upper body. Start with very small movements and use just the "pushing" motion.

Search for a rhythm that keeps the horse relaxed, letting the horse swing back into your hand with each rock (fig. 8.6). If you rock too hard, the horse will tense up, even if you don't see it. This is the part that takes a little practice. If you are doing it correctly, the horse's nose should be going in little circles. Imagine that if you put a magic marker in his mouth and hold a pad of paper to it, he would draw little circles on the pad: going clockwise on one side and counterclockwise on the other.

"Sneak up" on the horse with tiny little movements at first. Give your body some time to get used to it, and your mind some time to get out of the way.

3. Gently apply the "helping hand."

As you get the rhythm going and you feel the horse begin to relax into it, you can increase the movement a little. You may begin to use your helping hand on the hip to, well… help.

Develop the rhythm! You will find that every horse has his own individual rhythm. It helps to keep the image of a tub of water in mind. You are trying to slosh the water to create a wave that goes back and forth. Depending on the size of the tub and the amount of water, you will rock a little faster or a little slower. Gentle reminder: *Remember to breathe* and rock on!

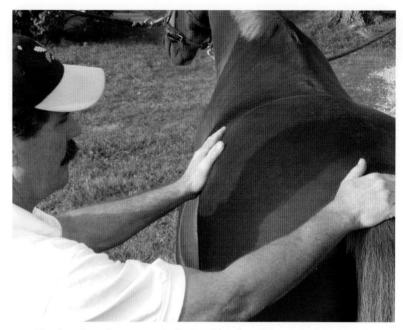

8.5 The hand on the sacrum is the "rocking hand," and the hand on the hip is the "helping hand."

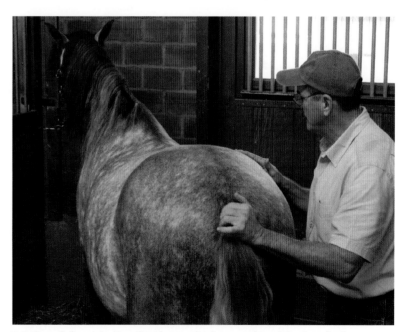

8.6 Search for a rhythm that keeps the horse relaxed, letting the horse swing back into your hand with each rocking motion.

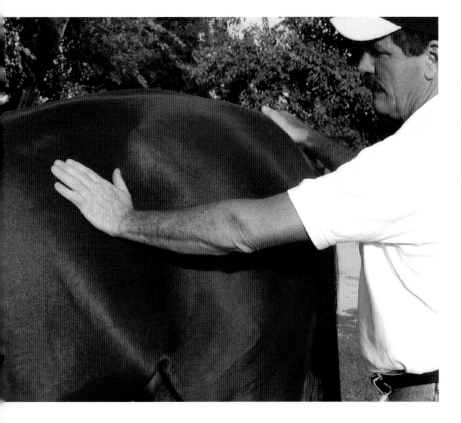

Keep moving forward, watching for "blinks" that will tell you if there is something on a spot that needs releasing. By watching the horse's responses, especially the eye, you can tell where there might be tension or blocked pain. You can also tell by the eye when he might be tensing, or relaxing and releasing. If you see the eye widen, or sense that he is tensing, soften the rocking slightly, giving him a chance to relax and release tension.

When he releases something you will feel him soften, and see the eye soften. Often you will see him lick and chew at the same time as he softens. When you get a release in one area, you can continue rocking, sliding your hand forward along each rib, all the way to the ribs behind the withers.

What Ifs?

■ *What if the horse stays rigid and his nose does not go in little circles?*

Not all horses are able to immediately translate movement in the hind end through their spine into the neck and head. Longstanding tension, back pain, or structural issues may make it difficult for him to relax, at first. It may also be that he is just not relaxed in general, or is distracted by other horses, and activity in the barn such as feeding. He also may be protecting an area of concern that you are touching during the exercise. In this case, *soften* the rocking slightly, but continue with gentle rocking for at least half a minute.

Some horses will try to resist relaxing, whether to protect an area of discomfort or because this rocking is new to them. If you stick

8.7 Once you have the horse rocking gently side to side, you can move the "helping hand" forward along the ribs.

4. Focus the movement on specific areas of the back.

Now that you have him rocking gently side to side, you can begin to focus movement on specific areas of the back with the helping hand. Each rib is attached to a corresponding vertebra. Rocking gently on a rib creates micro-movement in the corresponding vertebra, releasing tension in corresponding muscles and ligaments. You do this by sliding your helping hand forward with each "rock," and continuing rocking, along each rib, using the helping hand to focus the movement on any rib that corresponds to an area of that back that might be sore or stiff (fig. 8.7). You can spend a few "rocks" on each rib.

with it, though, and rock softly enough and long enough (this sounds familiar!) the horse will eventually give in and you may be surprised at the releases you get.

Note: This exercise will be easier if you are relaxed yourself. Make sure you aren't working too hard with your arms, and let the movement come from your waist and shoulders, with your knees slightly bent and elastic.

■ **What if the horse pins his ears or shows signs of agitation when I am on a particular spot?**

This can be a warning sign of pain or discomfort in this area, which means two things:

1. You need to back off, and…
2. You need to go back and help him release the pain.

Return to the last area on the horse where you worked with the horse feeling comfortable and *very* gently work your way toward the area of discomfort. Remember this is like peeling a layer of an onion. If you can gently peel the surface layer, often when you come back over that area the next time, it will be improved. As you peel away at your horse's tensions, you will eventually come to a place where this exercise is comfortable for the horse. If not, this may be an indication that a veterinarian needs to be consulted.

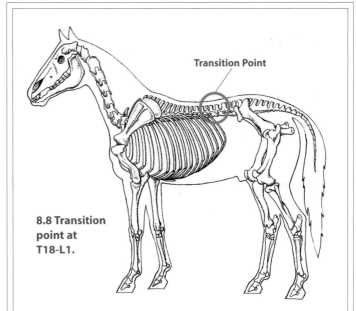

8.8 Transition point at T18-L1.

Transition Points of the Spine

The *transition point* where the thoracic spine (with corresponding ribs) ends and the lumbar spine begins (T18-L1) is a point at which muscle spasms often develop (fig. 8.8). These can be due to the effects of improper saddle fit or incorrect riding, but can also be due to an imbalance in the hind end caused by hock, stifle, or foot issues, especially when unilateral.

In general, the transition points between the different sections of the spine are areas at which tension often accumulates. You may have noticed that three of these other transition points—the *Poll-Atlas,* the *C7-T1,* and the *Sacroiliac*—are the key junctions that most affect performance.

Before you do this Technique, you may palpate down the top of the spine for knots or reactions, and focus the rocking on the ribs corresponding to those knots or reactions.

■ *How long should I do this?*

The best guideline is to let the horse's responses be your guide. If you reach a point where he is relaxed—lowers his head, finishes licking, chewing or yawning—then he may be done. When he seems stiff and his eyes and ears are tense, you should soften a little and continue rocking. If he fidgets, walks off, swishes his tail, and pins his ears, see the answer to the previous question.

Technique 2:
DORSAL ARCH

Before You Begin

GOAL: To create dorsal (upward) movement in the thoracic and lumbar vertebrae, encouraging the horse to "tuck in" his abdomen and arch his back in order to open up space between the *spinous processes* of these vertebrae.

RESULT: This active stretching movement releases pain and restriction in the back, causes greater flexibility in the back and pelvis, and improves ability to round the back and step under.

WHERE YOU WORK — ANATOMY

The focus of this Technique is also on the back from the withers to the tail, as well as the supporting muscles such as *abdominals, intercostals,* and

muscles deep inside the pelvic structure such as the *psoas* (fig. 8.9).

The lumbar spine acts as a "bridge" between the front and hind ends of the horse. The psoas are important muscles underneath the lumbar spine and pelvis. They are strong, short muscles that aid in tilting the pelvis, and are major stabilizers in the transference of power from the hind end to the body. They are often overlooked as they are hidden underneath everything and not easy to find and work on.

The *multifidi* muscles are mini-stabilizers woven through the vertebrae of the horse's spine. As these small, intertwined muscles are also hidden from view or touch, you can release them through an active stretch with the help of the horse.

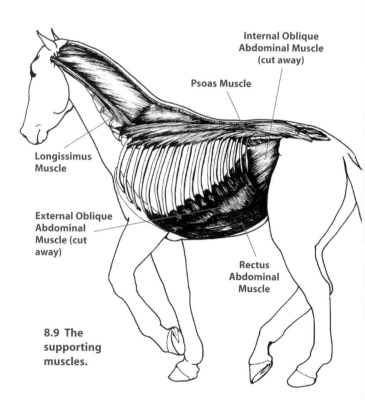

Internal Oblique
Abdominal Muscle
(cut away)

Psoas Muscle

Longissimus
Muscle

External Oblique
Abdominal
Muscle (cut
away)

Rectus
Abdominal
Muscle

8.9 The
supporting
muscles.

QUICK OVERVIEW: Step-by-Step

TECHNIQUE 2: DORSAL ARCH

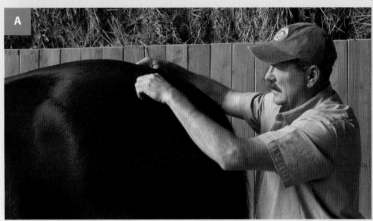

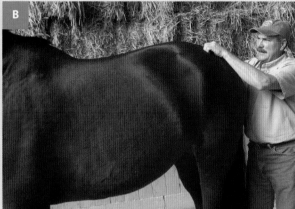

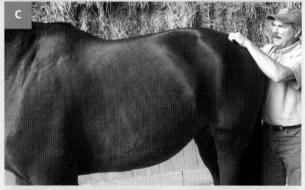

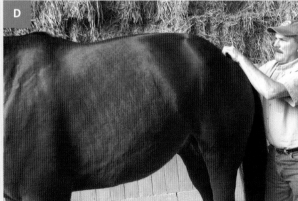

Step 1. Position yourself behind or slightly to the side of your horse's hind end, facing forward (A).

Step 2. Bring your fingertips together or use something hard and smooth, such as a plastic pen cap, and push down on the gluteal muscle either side of the sacrum, behind the high point of the croup (B).

Step 3. Pull back toward the poverty groove as you push your hands down (C).

Step 4. When the horse starts to arch his back, adjust the pressure to control whether he arches less, or more (D).

Step 5. Step back and watch for signs of release.

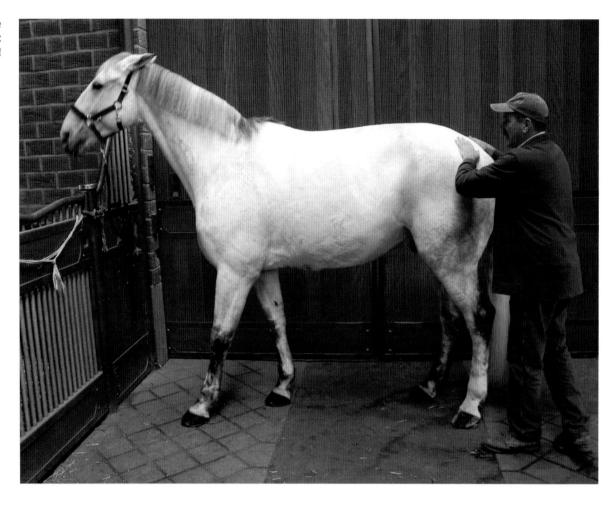

RELEASING TENSION: THE EFFECTS

Tension accumulated here over time can lead to a stiff, "cold" back that becomes rigid and inhibits the horse's ability to move freely and efficiently. "Opening" the vertebrae by encouraging the horse to arch his back up stretches and releases tension in the muscles of the back, enabling them to stretch and contract efficiently. This allows the horse to swing in the back, round it, and step under himself.

The *Dorsal Arch* exercise also actively engages abdominals and psoas muscles supporting the muscles of the back from below. Both the psoas and abdominal muscles are needed to tilt the pelvis and enable the horse to step under. And, as I've said before, the psoas muscles are also major stabilizers in the transference of power from the hind end to the body. They can become restricted in movement and end up doing either too much "stabilizing" and less "aiding," or may become overstressed and freeze up and stop working altogether. The good news is that with the *Hind End Techniques* you have been using, both *From the Top* and *From the Bottom,* you have already been loosening and activating these important muscles (see chapter 7). Asking them to move now is going to help even more.

Once the back is flexible and subtle, these muscle groups, along with the abdominals and *longissimus dorsi,* can do their job of balancing both ends of the horse and enabling the horse to develop "positive" self-carriage while carrying the rider.

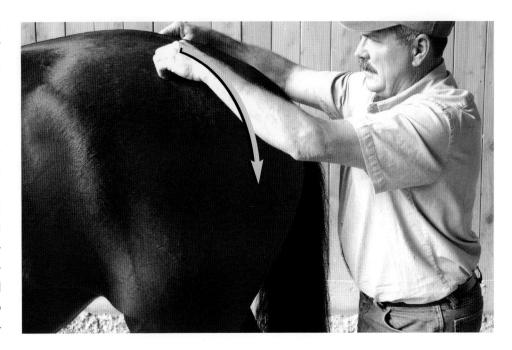

8.13 Push down and drag.

Safety Note: *As you will be standing directly behind the horse for this Technique you need to pay especially close attention to the horse's ears, or other signs of discomfort in the horse as you do this (fig. 8.12). If the horse's ears start to flatten, stop!*

The horse's response to pressure should be a *reflex* reaction, *not* a *pain* reaction. If this Technique hurts the horse it shouldn't be done.

When working on a unfamiliar horse or if you suspect the horse might still be sore and there's a possibility he could kick, stack two bales of hay between you and the horse.

Technique 2 in More Detail

In the *Lateral Rocking* exercise (p. 143) you released tension in muscles around the horse's spine by creating lateral movement. Now you want to create dorsal (upward) movement in the spine.

This very effective Technique is the only one you will use that requires active movement from the horse. You use reflex points to encourage the horse to contract the abdominal muscles and arch the back. For this reason, the exercise is sometimes referred to as "horse sit-ups."

1. Position yourself.

Stand behind or slightly off to the side of the horse's hind end. Bring your fingertips together to form a strong point of contact. Place them on the gluteal muscle on either side of the sacrum, *behind* the high point of the croup. If you push down on or in front of the croup, the horse will flex the back *downward*—not what you are looking for here.

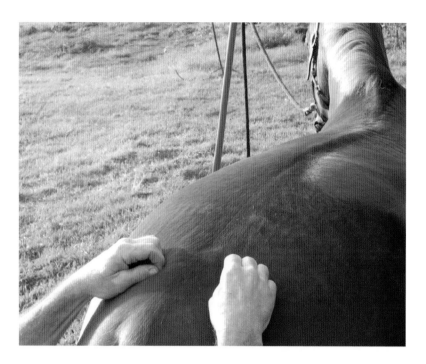

8.14 Start behind the croup and draw your hands down toward you.

your hands down toward you watch for the horse to start to raise his back a little bit (fig. 8.14). When he does this you can increase—or decrease—pressure (use just enough) to get the horse to tuck the pelvis and arch the back. You can control how much he raises his back this way.

Safety Note: *Watch the horse's ears as you draw your fingers back across the gluteals. If his ears go flat, STOP!*

If his ears flatten or he is uncomfortable with this, it is likely he has sore or sensitive gluteal muscles. In some cases, the horse can have issues with the back that make it uncomfortable for him to arch it, but in most cases, it is sensitivity in the gluteal muscles that causes this reaction.

At first you might think that this is hurting or bothering the horse, but if you step back to see what the horse's response will be, you will find that in most cases it is a relief for the horse to release this tension in the spine.

Tips

- I have found that many students, when they reach this point, have difficulty getting the horse to arch the back because up until now their attention has been on more subtle aspects of interaction, and their intention has been not to hurt the horse. No matter how hard they push, some of them cannot get the horse to go away from the pressure and arch the back. Not that you're going to hurt the horse, but it helps to change mental gears and have the *intention* to get the horse to move away

2. Draw your hands downward.

Push down with the tips of your fingers, using a fair amount of pressure—*lemon* or even *lime*—and draw your fingertips firmly straight back toward the poverty groove across the muscles to either side of the sacrum (fig. 8.13). As you draw

Dorsal Arch

A "Morning Stretch" for the Horse

When done correctly, this Technique seems to elicit the same reaction that we have when we stretch and twist our back first thing in the morning. This is not a very scientific observation, but that's the feeling I get.

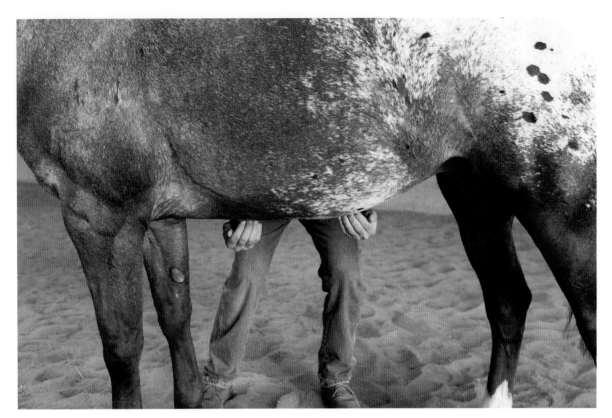

8.15 Use your fingertips or nails on the belly to ask the horse to lift.

from the pressure you are putting on his rump. This pressure initiates a reflex reaction, and unless the horse flattens his ears, it's not hurting him—it's helping him.

■ A little *Lateral Rocking* again after the *Dorsal Arch* will loosen up the back even more.

■ It's better not to perform this exercise more than two or three times in one session and no more than twice per week. Muscles that have been inactive or restricted can become tender.

■ In addition, since the success of this Technique depends on the horse's ability to react to

Kissing Spines

If your horse has been diagnosed by a veterinarian to have actual "kissing spines" or spinous process impingement, it would be wise to consult your vet prior to performing this Technique. While this Technique can help to open or widen the spaces between the vertebrae, it would be a good idea to check to make sure there is nothing that could be aggravated.

manipulation of the reflex zone, you will want to be sure not to numb the response by performing the exercise too frequently and desensitizing the horse.

What Ifs?

■ **What if the horse does not arch his back or show any reaction at all?**

Since you are using a reflex point to affect this reaction, there is no rule of thumb on how much reaction an individual horse will show. Some horses are very sensitive, some can seem downright numb to the manipulation.

Be sure to use enough pressure. It's easy to underestimate the amount of pressure needed, depending on the horse. If needed, use something harder than your fingertips. A quarter coin held between the fingers of each hand can help you get the needed pressure to get a reaction, and doesn't cost very much. If all fails, try the "Belly Lift" exercise described on this page.

■ **What if I hear "popping" noises as he arches his back?**

This is a good thing. Vertebrae that are stiff or haven't moved upward, or arched, for a while often make a popping sound, similar to the sound we get when we crack our kuckles, when you arch the horse's back. Large *release responses* usually accompany popping, along with increased movement and suppleness in the back.

■ **What if the horse is overly reactive and flinches or flattens his ears when I press down?**

The horse may be sensitive due to a number of reasons, either naturally sensitive, or sore. Simply go lighter, soften your touch or find a point to start that's a bit farther back toward the poverty groove.

■ **I have always used the Belly-Lift Exercise to get my horse to arch his back. Is this wrong?**

I prefer this gluteal method as the horse is encouraged to tilt the pelvis more, but the *Belly Lift* works well to arch the back, and you're not standing directly behind the horse. It is a good alternative to the *Dorsal Arch* when the horse does not react at all to manipulation of the reflex zone on the gluteals.

The *Belly Lift* is done by standing facing the side of the horse as if looking across his back. Press up against the centerline of the belly with your fingertips and encourage the horse to raise his back (fig. 8.15). It helps to wiggle your fingertips and actually "tickle" the belly up.

Safety Note: It is still important to watch the horse's ears for discomfort during the Belly Lift, because he can cow-kick to the side almost as easily and quickly as kicking to the rear.

PART THREE

Addressing Performance Issues

GENERAL PROBLEMS, INDIVIDUAL BREEDS, AND PRE-EVENT BODYWORK

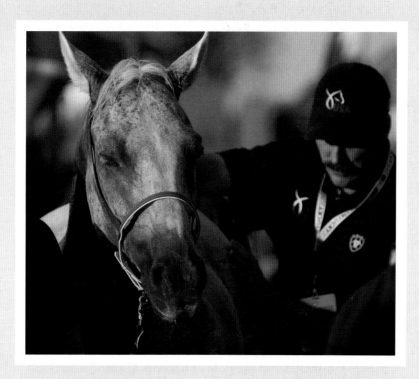

CHAPTER 9

Performance Problems

Primary Issues vs Secondary Issues

Much of what you work on in the body is secondary to, or is being caused by a *primary* issue or issues. This can be a *direct* issue such as a poorly fitting saddle, or *compensation* for a physical issue, such as foot pain.

When the horse compensates for discomfort that has been created by a *primary* issue, *secondary* issues are created—pain, tension, and restriction—that affect performance. Releasing this pain, tension, and restriction will improve your horse's performance, but only when you can determine what the primary issue is will you also be able to prevent the return of these secondary issues. In many cases, you will also be able to prevent the primary issue from becoming a serious physical or veterinary issue.

Below are some examples of *primary issues:*

Foot and Lower Leg Pain

- Pain in the lower leg due to inflammation of the splint bone(s), ligaments, tendons, knee, pastern joints, stifles, and hocks.

- Pain in the foot due to thrush, laminitis, inflammation of the coffin joint, navicular syndrome, general tender-footedness, or improper shoeing.

Saddle and Other Tack

- Saddle fit: tree, padding, gullet, length, all incorrect size.

- Saddle condition: tree broken or twisted, flocking or padding distorted, wear or damage.

- Auxiliary tack: improper fit or use.

- Bit: improper fit, adjustment, or use.

Dental Issues

- Floating.

- Imbalanced teeth.

Riding Style

- Unbalanced riding can cause some muscles to become over-stressed and others to become under-developed.

Conformational Issues

- Crooked feet or legs.

- Long or short in the back.

- How he's "put together."

Tension in the body can also develop from the effects of the horse's daily work. Muscle tension patterns arise from repeated contractions, and when some muscles end up doing more work than others, imbalances occur. (This is why it's important to condition and ride the horse in such a way so he develops fitness in a natural and balanced manner.)

And finally, as explained earlier (see "Where You Start Work—Symmetry and Asymmetry in the Horse," p. 23), unilateral tension can develop as a result of the horse's natural asymmetry or his tendency to have a stronger or more predominant side. This imbalance may be emphasized with work and over time can create larger imbalances that contribute to physical issues or lameness.

Finding the Culprit

When determining possible primary issues, bear in mind that the horse is a herd animal that instinctively does his best *not* to show outward signs of pain or weakness (why it is often difficult to accurately evaluate lameness). Consequently, primary issues can go undetected for ages and the longer this happens, the more tension accumulates. Sometimes, determining if there is a primary issue and what it might be is rather like putting together the pieces of a puzzle.

Residual Muscle Tension Patterns

Often the underlying problem is no longer an issue or has been resolved, yet the horse still suffers from the residual effects of compensation. Or, to put it another way: Even when the pain or primary issue that created muscle tension patterns in the body has gone, the muscle tension patterns can remain, especially when the tension has been around for a long time. In this case, you can often bring about a permanent improvement in performance through bodywork.

When the primary issue is not resolved, compensatory muscle tension patterns will return even *after* you have helped the horse to release them. In this case, identifying and eliminating the primary issue is most helpful.

The more data or information you can gather, the better your chances are of finding what might be causing the pain and tension as well as being able to do something about it.

Here are things to consider when looking for the culprit:

Diagonals

One of the most valuable pieces of information that you can gather from working on your horse's body is which fore-hind *diagonal* is holding the most tension. This helps you to make sense of the way your horse goes; which his predominant lead is; where his tension accumulates; where his primary issues might be; and where to keep an eye out for future problems.

Pain vs. Restriction

Some performance problems are related more to *pain* or *discomfort* while others more to *stiffness and restriction*. Generally, stiffness is an older issue—or one that has developed over time—and pain is related to something that is bothering the horse at the moment. Knowing which could be causing your performance problem can help you determine the primary issue. See the charts: figs 9.1 A & B.

Note: These charts are based on my experience only, and large amounts of money should not be bet on it!

It Is Almost Never Just "One Thing"!

As different parts of the horse are interconnected, so one area of tension, or even a lameness, is connected to another area. So it helps to give attention to the front end when focusing on a possible hind-end issue, and to give attention to the sacrum and hind end when focusing on a possible front-end issue.

Other Considerations

While working on the horse take note of where the horse has the most trouble releasing. For example, when he releases easily behind but has difficulty releasing the scapula or upper neck, poll, or atlas on one side, your focus should be on the *front end*. When the front-end releases go easily yet you find the hind-leg release on one side to be difficult, a stifle point very tender, or the sacrum "clamped down" at the *Under-the-Tail Points,* the focus should be on the *hind end*. Whatever area is the most difficult to release often indicates the place where the primary issue might be. This will help you narrow down where the culprit might be hiding.

Look at the whole horse, and pay attention to the connections pointed out in this book between hind and front ends, including the relationship between the front to hind end diagonals:

- Tension in the atlas is connected to tension in the sacrum.

- Often tension in the poll on one side is connected to a muscle spasm in the gluteal muscle at the hip joint on the *opposite* hind diagonal.

- Tension in the Neck-Shoulder-Withers Junction (under the scapula) is connected to tension in the lumbar area, pelvis, and sacrum.

- Horses with hock issues frequently have excessive soreness or tension in the hamstring muscles.

- Stifle issues or soreness in the stifles, often goes along with excessive soreness or tension in the groin and lumbar areas.

Is My Horse's Problem Caused by...

PAIN OR RESTRICTION?

Performance Problem	Restriction	Pain
1. Lead Change Problems	X	**X**
2. Not Using His Back	X	**X**
3. Resisting the Bit	X	**X**
4. Heavy on the Forehand	**X**	X
5. Not Stepping Under Behind	**X**	X
6. Holds Head Flat, Crooked	**X**	X
7. Intermittent Lameness	**X**	X
8. Does Not Move Out with Front Legs	**X**	X
9. Choppy, Short-Strided	**X**	X
10. "Girthy"		**X**
11. Head-Shy	X	**X**
12. Ewe-Necked, Hollow-Backed	**X**	X
13. Doesn't Bend in the Body	**X**	X
14. Formerly Agile, Now Lazy	**X**	X
15. Bucking, Rushing		**X**
16. Hitches Leg or Drags Toe	X	**X**

A PRIMARY OR SECONDARY ISSUE?

Performance Problem	Possible Primary Issue	Possible Secondary Issue
1. Lead Change Problems	**X**	X
2. Sore or Rigid Back	**X**	X
3. Resisting the Bit	**X**	X
4. Heavy on the Forehand	X	**X**
5. Not Stepping Under Behind	X	**X**
6. Holds Head Flat, Crooked	X	**X**
7. Intermittent Lameness	**X**	X
8. Does Not Move Out with Front Legs	X	**X**
9. Choppy, Short-Strided	X	**X**
10. "Girthy"	**X**	
11. Head-Shy	**X**	X
12. Ewe-Necked, Hollow-Backed	X	**X**
13. Doesn't Bend Body	X	**X**
14. Formerly Agile, Now Lazy	X	**X**
15. Bucking, Rushing	**X**	
16. Hitches Leg or Drags Toe	**X**	X

9.1 A & B If both columns are marked with an X, both may be an issue. A bold X indicates that the issue is more likely. A light X indicates less likely. These charts are not meant to diagnose actual physical problems. That is the job of your vet—you should call him when there is any doubt about whether there could be a serious physical problem.

Individual Performance Problems

■ The one thing that should be done during the course of addressing any performance problem, whether you are focusing on the *back*, the *hind end* or the *front end,* and that is to release tension in the poll and atlas. It helps to release tension in the entire body, makes the rest of the releases easier and makes them last longer. Everything connects to the poll and atlas.

Note: When addressing any of the performance problems listed below, remember you are often addressing the horse'e way of compensating for an underlying problem.

PERFORMANCE PROBLEMS

Here is a list of the problems that are covered on the pages ahead with suggested Techniques. These are listed alphabetically together with the page number where they are addressed.

1. LEAD PROBLEMS

The horse has difficulty picking up, or staying on, a particular canter lead.

Possible Primary Issues

This is one of the most common performance problems I come across.

When a horse has difficulty going on a particular lead, it's possible he is uncomfortable in this direction, which suggests a *primary problem:* A lameness issue usually shows up first at the trot. When this is the case, a veterinary exam is indicated.

When a primary issue is not serious enough to create lameness, it can still bother the horse enough so he *compensates* for it by staying on one particular lead rather than the other. Tension patterns develop in the compensatory muscles, creating an imbalance in the way the horse moves.

The primary issue could be in either the front or hind end of the horse. Often, but not always, this distinction can be felt by the rider, giving a first indication of where to start looking.

Front End

Some examples of primary issues in the front end are: pain from an abscess, and inflammation of a splint bone or coffin joint that has been building but has not yet created an observable lameness. In compensation, the horse develops tension in muscles that connect the affected foreleg to the neck, atlas and poll. Prolonged contraction of these muscles, for example, the *brachiocephalicus* or *omotransversarius* (fig. 6.2, p. 64) will cause soreness and unilateral restrictions in the neck, atlas and poll.

Furthermore, when unilateral tension on the atlas and poll causes them to become tight or restricted to one side—or misaligned—it affects the function of not only the front end, but the hind end as well. For example, an atlas that is misaligned, or restricted by contraction on one side, can cause muscle spasms in the gluteal muscles at the hip joint on the diagonal hind leg. When the tension in the poll and atlas is cleared up, the spasm at the gluteal improves, or often disappears completely.

When the horse compensates for foot or foreleg discomfort long enough, a restriction in movement also starts to show up in the Neck-Trunk (C7-T1) Junction as he tries to get away from the discomfort in the affected leg with each step. This restriction will create further lead-change issues as the muscles that connect the front end to the hind end, such as the *longissimus dorsi* and the *iliocostal* muscles (see fig. 7.9, p. 110) develop tension patterns that make it even more uncomfortable for him to canter on one lead.

How to Address

Techniques to use to release tension in the *front end*:

Techniques (Front End)	Page
Poll and Atlas Releases (Head Up, Head Down)	*pp. 45 and 51*
Lateral Flexion	*p. 33*
Scapula Releases	*pp. 62 and 80*
C7-T1 Release	*p. 92*

Hind End

Common primary issues in the hind end often have to do with the hocks or stifles. Some of the muscles the horse uses to compensate for discomfort in the hocks or stifles include the groin, hamstring, lumbar and gluteal muscles. When these muscles put enough tension on the sacrum, especially unilaterally, it creates torque on the sacroiliac joint. In my experience, when the sacroiliac becomes "torqued," it affects muscles of the hind end, which can affect the lead change.

Note: This type of tension or torque of the sacrum can also originate from work or training (see Primary vs. Secondary Issues, p. 160.)

When you release tension on the sacrum, you release tension in the muscles of the hind end. You can get further release of tension in muscles that may be contributing to the lead problem, such as the gluteal spasm at the hip joint (see "Other Considerations", p. 162), by moving the hind limbs through a range of movement in a relaxed state.

How to Address

Techniques to use to release tension in the *hind end*:

Techniques (Hind End)	Page
Poll and Atlas Releases (Head Up, Head Down)	*pp. 45 and 51*
Hind End Release Points	*p. 111*
Hind Leg Releases	*p. 125*

2. SORE OR RIGID BACK

Possible Primary Issues

A sore back is one of those whole-body issues. The horse has to be able to use his back fully in order for the front and hind ends to work together—in all gaits. Sometimes, the back itself is the primary issue, and sometimes there may be another cause—in the front or hind end. In either case, when the back ceases to function naturally, it affects the functioning of the body as a whole.

It's important the primary issue is determined. Otherwise the soreness will return, no matter how much bodywork you do on the back.

Common primary issues:

- Prior injury.
- Poor saddle fit.
- Compensation for feet or leg issues—front and hind.
- Improper riding and conditioning.
- Dental issues.

The more longstanding the soreness in the back, the more rigid the back becomes as circulation is cut off and the muscles atrophy. Often, there may no longer be soreness because the muscles of the back may completely "shut down" and nerves damaged.

In some cases, the primary cause may have been removed and no longer be an issue, yet the back has shut down and remains rigid as a result of the prior issue. However, once you have done the work to free up the back, it may remain relatively loose and begin to function naturally to some degree.

Note: *The back is not just "something you sit on" but an essential part of equine locomotion. Tension or restriction in the back prevents proper movement and natural gaits.*

How to Address

Techniques to use:

Techniques	Page
Poll and Atlas Releases (Head Up, Head Down)	*pp. 45 and 51*
Scapula Releases	*pp. 62 and 80*
Hind End Points and Leg Releases	*pp. 111 and 125*
C7-T1 Release	*p. 92*
Lateral Rocking	*p. 143*
Dorsal Arch	*p. 152*

Often simply doing some *Lateral Rocking,* then the *Dorsal Arch* will loosen up the back and you will see an improvement. However, for deeper or more longstanding back problems you will need to first thoroughly loosen up the front and hind ends *then* work toward the middle with the *Back Releases.* Both ends of the horse have to be loose in order for the back to let go.

Remember that if the back is sore there may be a primary issue that needs to be dealt with. Find the primary issue, and keep the back released and loose on a regular basis.

3. RESISTING THE BIT

Possible Primary Issues

Often the horse resists the bit to avoid pain or discomfort in the upper neck, atlas, poll or TMJ. For example, the horse will pull against the bit to avoid pain in the poll and upper neck when asked to flex in this area. I discussed earlier how a front-limb issue may cause pain in the poll. A primary issue in the front limb may not be bad enough to cause the horse to be lame, but compensating for discomfort here will over time create tension in the poll, upper neck, and possibly the TMJ. This can cause the horse to resist the bit.

The horse will also resist the bit if the TMJ itself becomes sore due to dental issues.

When the horse resists the bit as he is asked to get "under himself," it's possible there is an issue behind and the horse is avoiding using his hind end. He wants to stay on the forehand so leans on the bit. This is discussed further under "Heavy on the Forehand".

How to Address
Techniques to use:

Techniques	Page
Poll and Atlas Releases (Head Up, Head Down)	*pp. 45 and 51*
Scapula Releases	*pp. 62 and 80*

4. HEAVY ON THE FOREHAND

Possible Primary Issues

The horse will often load the forehand when there is pain or discomfort somewhere in the hind limbs or muscles of the hind end, as he tries to keep the weight off there. When he resists the bit while being asked to collect and use the hind end, this may be the case. Releasing tension in the hind end allows it to work more efficiently and often relieves the horse's need to load the front end. If there is a serious primary or veterinary issue in the hind end, the horse may continue to load the front end. If this performance issue persists, it may be wise to have a veterinarian look at the horse.

How to Address
Techniques to use:

Techniques	Page
Hind End Release Points	*p. 111*
Hind Leg Releases	*p. 125*

When the horse is heavy on the forehand, I usually first look to the hind end to help with the problem.

In addition to the *Hind End Points and Hind Leg Releases,* loosening up the back with *Lateral Rocking* and *Dorsal Arch* makes it easier for the horse to use the hind end properly once it is working better. To further release tension in the *longissimus dorsi* muscle, also release tension in the C7–T1 Junction.

5. NOT STEPPING UNDER BEHIND

Also: Not using the hind end; lack of impulsion; not rounding in the back.

Possible Primary Issues

When looking at an inability to step under himself or "round" his back, you are usually looking at a horse that is *contracted* on the topline.

For the horse to be able to use his hind end effectively, he has to be able to use the whole body together. He must be able to round in the back, to step under his body with his hind legs and use the hind end. An inability to do this can be the result of overwork behind, and is often coupled with the horse being collected too much in the front end.

Other primary issues can be poor saddle fit, soft-tissue, or joint issues: front end or hind end. Whatever the cause, tension or torque on the *sacrum* will end up being a key factor in the horse being unable to step under and drive from behind.

How to Address

Techniques to use:

Techniques	Page
Poll and Atlas Releases (Head Up, Head Down)	*pp. 45 and 51*
Hind End Release Points	*p. 111*
Hind Leg Releases	*p. 125*
Lateral Rocking	*p. 143*
Dorsal Arch	*p. 152*

Your strategy is to release tension in the back *and* at both ends: The easiest way to begin releasing tension in the sacrum is to release tension in the poll and atlas. Once the topline is released, the back can do its job and the whole body will be able to work together thus allowing the horse to use the hind end effectively.

Unless the area around the atlas is too sore or sensitive to work with, start there because releasing tension in the atlas begins the process of release in the sacrum and hind end. When you arrive at the hind end, start with the *Release Points* to see what you get.

Pay close attention to the hamstrings creating torque or tension on the sacrum. Overwork behind and hock issues often have to do with over-contraction of the hamstrings.

Once you have loosened up the horse using *Release Points,* go on to the *Leg Releases,* paying close attention to where he has the most restriction, discomfort, or gives the biggest releases. This is where you will focus on releasing tension.

Also pay close attention to the lumbar area.

Often, it will not show any signs of soreness or sensitivity, but might be stiff and immobile. Restriction in the sacrolumbar area blocks the chain of movement from the hind end through to the back, affecting the horse's ability to use the whole body.

After the *Leg Releases,* spend more time than you would think on *Lateral Rocking.* It may take a while for the horse to stop guarding his lower back, but when he does, the releases will be large. Follow this up with *Dorsal Arch.*

6. HOLDS HEAD FLAT, CROOKED, OR TO THE SIDE

Also: Resists the bit to one side; bends neck better in one direction than the other.

Possible Primary Issues

Excessive unilateral tension in muscles and ligaments in the poll and neck can lead to bending and unilateral resistance issues. A muscle that is constantly contracted (e.g. *brachiocephalic*) on one side can cause crookedness in the neck.

As explained earlier, this contraction can come from front foot or leg pain or discomfort, usually on the same side in which the horse will not bend, or the side he resists the bit.

In addition, horses are like humans in that they usually have a stronger and more predominant side. Thus, they can develop unilateral tension patterns over time that will manifest as performance issues such as this. Regular releasing of these tension patterns will help keep the horse even.

During the *Lateral Cervical Flexion Technique,* look for certain places where there is restriction of movement or less flexibility, especially the difference from one side to the other. This is where you want to ask the horse to release tension. Remember to start releasing tension on the easier (opposite) side first and to work on both sides of the neck.

How to Address

Techniques to use:

Techniques	Page
Poll and Atlas Releases (Head Up, Head Down)	*pp. 45 and 51*
Lateral Flexion	*p. 33*
Scapula Releases	*pp. 62 and 80*
C7-T1 Release	*p. 92*

By focusing on the poll and atlas, and the scapula at the *C7-T1 Junction,* you are working on the attachments on both ends of two major muscles (*brachiocephalic and omotransverse*) involved. This makes it easier and more effective when you get to the area of restricted movement—the upper neck. Here you will focus on releasing tension with a very light touch.

Lateral movement in the relaxed *Head Up* position will also help with this problem.

Note: Remember that any time you are having trouble working on an area, or the horse is uncomfortable where you are working, go to the opposite side and release the tension there first. You will find that having worked on the easier side first, the horse will have released much of the tension on the difficult side. *Don't attack the problem area. Go where it is easier first.*

Tension in the poll and atlas is related to most performance issues. Releasing tension here makes the release of tension in other areas of the body easier, and last longer.

7. INTERMITTENT FRONT END "LAMENESS"

Possible Primary Issues

In my experience, this often happens after the horse has had a front-leg lameness of some sort for an extended period of time. After it has been treated or has healed, the horse will sometimes continue to be intermittently lame and sound, in some cases, for months. The longer the horse has been lame on the leg, the longer this subsequent intermittent lameness lasts.

Compensation for the lameness over a long period of time has created muscle tension patterns that put unilateral tension, or torque on the *C7-T1 Junction.* Once the primary initial lameness is gone, this torque remains and shows up as intermittent lameness until it releases. It may relax and let go over time if allowed, but it makes sense to try to help the horse release it sooner.

How to Address

I have found that releasing tension in the *C7–T1 Junction* where the last vertebra of the neck joins the first vertebra of the body very often helps this, or even clears it up.

After the poll, atlas, and vertebrae of the neck have been released, it is important to release as much tension in the *Neck-Withers C7-T1 Junction* as possible with the *Scapula Releases:* One way to help with this when *Releasing Down and Forward* is to ask the horse to relax the leg in front across the midline. If there is torque in the C7-T1 Junction, the horse will be uncomfortable doing this. The remedy is to back off while supporting the leg, and allow the horse to relax in as comfortable a position close to this as possible. Wait for the release, and watch for the signs.

After this release go to the *C7-T1 Release.* Go slowly and allow the horse to relax into it. If you feel you have got some release here, check back to see if there is any improvement in releasing the leg forward across the midline. If there is, you will probably have made some improvement in the intermittent lameness issue.

Techniques to use:

Techniques	Page
Poll and Atlas Releases (Head Up, Head Down)	*pp. 45 and 51*
Scapula Releases	*pp. 62 and 80*
C7-T1 Release	*p. 92*

Note: *The best thing for the horse after a big release is movement: turnout, an easy walk or hack on a loose rein, or hand-walking. Let the horse rest overnight, and look for an improvement the next day.*

8. DOES NOT EXTEND OUT WITH FRONT LEGS

Also: Restricted in shoulders; short-strided in front.

Possible Primary Issues

Restriction in the front end can:

1. Develop over time simply from work.
2. Be the result of working with front foot pain.
3. Result from the horse trying to stay off the hind end.

The most common in my experience are the first two examples, although any work you can do on the hind end that makes it easier for the horse to stay off the forehand will help keep the front end loose. I compare the effect that front-end restriction has on performance, to asking a swimmer to swim a mile with a stiff neck or a knot between the shoulder blades.

All the components of the front end—the neck and head, withers, shoulders, and legs—need to work together to keep the front end loose and functioning efficiently.

The horse's head and neck are important for movement of the front legs, and to balance the whole horse in movement. The soft-tissue connection of the scapula to the horse's body needs to be loose and flexible. The withers and trunk are the anchor for this support, and for moving the horse forward.

Case History

I remember the first time I realized how effective these Front End Techniques can be in simply improving performance. After I'd worked on a young lady's equitation horse on the circuit in Wellington, Florida, she took the horse out for a hack. During the session I hadn't seen anything that stood out as being a problem—only the usual tension accumulated in the course of doing his job. I did get a nice surprise, though, when she returned with a big smile on her face. "Wow! That's the first time I've ever really seen his front feet while trotting out!"

Sometimes we don't realize how much restriction accumulates in the horse until we release accumulated it.

How to Address

Techniques to use:

Techniques	Page
Poll and Atlas Releases (Head Up, Head Down)	*pp. 45 and 51*
Scapula Releases	*pp. 62 and 80*
C7-T1 Release	*p. 92*
Withers Wiggle	*p. 100*
Lateral Cervical Flexion	*p. 33*

All of the *Front End Techniques* will help keep these essential components moving freely. Working on the poll and atlas releases tension in large muscles that insert at the other end on the forearm, and on the withers. *Scapula Releases* help with extension and suspension (shock absorption). C7–T1 Releases are the key to keeping the *Neck-Shoulder-Withers Junction* free. As you loosen up all these areas, the muscles and tendons of the leg also release tension. All this allows for better extension of the front legs, and for all of the components of this junction to work together.

9. CHOPPY GAIT; SHORT-STRIDED; HARD TO SIT AT THE TROT

Possible Primary Issues
Some horses are naturally choppy, short-strided, and hard to sit at the trot due to their conformation or body type. These horses can be helped to loosen up to some degree using the Techniques taught in this book.

When this is a performance rather than a conformational problem, it will most likely have to do with a long-term primary issue. Stiffness caused by the horse compensating over a long period for any of the possible primary issues listed above, whether in the front end, hind end or back will eventually take away his shock-absorbing ability.

How to Address
This is basically the same principle as with the *front end* as described on p. 170, except you are releasing tension in the junctions of *both* the hind limbs and the body, and the front limbs and the body. You then connect the two by releasing tension in the back.

Releasing tension in the two junctions where limbs join the body will help the horse relax during movement, provide suspension and allow relaxed swinging of the limbs and back.

Techniques to use:

Techniques	Page
Scapula Releases	*pp. 62 and 80*
C7-T1 Release	*p. 92*
Hind Leg Releases	*p. 125*
Lateral Rocking	*p. 143*
Dorsal Arch	*p. 152*

10. "GIRTHY" OR "CINCHY"

Possible Primary Issues
A "girthy" or "cinchy" reaction is sometimes to pain in the pectoral muscles at the girth line. This may come from over-girthing the saddle, or from work or training that is requiring excessive use of these muscles.

There is also a correlation between pain here and front foot pain. Often horses have pain here when they have an abscess, splint-bone pain, coffin-joint pain, or chronic navicular syndrome, for example. In my experience "girthiness" is a reliable indicator that there may be something going on in the lower leg at the time. You can determine by palpation on which side the reaction is greater thus indicating where the issue is.

As mentioned above, this reaction in the pectoral muscles at the girth can be a sign of current discomfort in the foot and leg—as opposed to tension or stiffness in the poll or upper neck, which may remain after a past foot issue has been resolved.

How to Address
Techniques to use:

Techniques	Page
Poll and Atlas Releases (Head Up, Head Down)	*pp. 45 and 51*
Scapula Releases	*pp. 62 and 80*
C7-T1 Release	*p. 92*
Lateral Rocking	*p. 143*

While holding the leg up during the *Scapula Release—Down and Back* take the time to gently stroke *(effleurage)* the pectorals under the leg from behind the sternum back to the abdomen. You can also do this while the leg is resting on the ground in the back position, and resting on the ground in the forward position. After doing the *Leg Release* forward, gently ask for a release out to the side (laterally). This will help to elongate the pectorals in a relaxed state. Then get under the scapula to release the C7–T-1 Junction. Here at the sternum is where some of these muscles originate.

As an added bonus, *Lateral Rocking* of the ribs will help to relax the abdomen, at the other end of the pectorals. However, the "girthyness" or pain in the pectorals will return until the issue with the foot or leg is resolved, so it is in your (and the horse's) interest to find and treat the primary problem.

11. HEAD-SHY
Also: Sensitive to touch on poll and ears.

Possible Primary Issues
In my experience, 95 percent of head-shy horses are that way because of pain and tension in the poll and atlas.

There are many things that may be creating pain or tension in the poll and atlas. Sore front feet and dental issues are two of the most common. Back soreness can cause tension just behind the poll and on top of the atlas, and I believe that mental stress and tension can also develop into "headaches" in the horse. Some horses and breeds that are more high strung than others have trouble relaxing tension there once it has accumulated. If a horse is head-shy, it's a 99 percent chance that he will need work, so releasing tension there can be one of the most rewarding things you can do for the horse.

How to Address
Techniques to use:

Techniques	Page
Poll and Atlas Releases (Head Up, Head Down)	*pp. 45 and 51*
Scapula and Under Scapula Releases	*pp. 62, 80 and 92*
Hind End Release Points	*p. 104*

The *Poll and Atlas Releases* are the key to releasing tension and relieving pain there, but aren't always the easiest things to do with a head-shy horse. The key to doing them is to keep the horse relaxed, and to stay as light as possible starting out. You may even want to start with *air gap* pressure or an *"extended air gap"* of as much as 4 to 5 inches. Once the horse realizes that he is not being forced, and that it feels good, it will be easier to work with him.

Another good alternative is to do the *Scapula Releases* first. This is generally easier for the horse in this situation, and even the smallest release will often break the ice and get enough endorphins going to make the next steps a little easier. If you can get the horse to relax through even a tiny bit of *Lateral Cervical Flexion* in the poll area, the horse will relax enough for you to do a little more, then a little more. Have patience, and from there you may be able to work gently up the neck toward the poll.

12. EWE-NECKED; HOLLOW-BACKED

Possible Primary Issues

This is a demonstration of how the whole body needs *to be able* to work together. A ewe-necked carriage develops over time as a result of the horse not using the muscles of the back and hind end properly. Overdeveloped lower neck muscles, insufficient development of back muscles, and weakened hind end muscles result. Not stepping under behind, a hollowed back and often short-ened strides round out this picture. The muscles of the back become stiff and atrophied, the horse becomes short-strided as the front and hind ends

have to work independently. Pain, as in the back, can cause the horse to carry his head in the air, and not use his hind end properly.

Releasing the muscles of the neck, lower neck, and the sacrolumbar junction—along with proper conditioning and riding—enables the horse to begin to use his body as a whole. Regular bodywork and proper conditioning and riding over time will help the horse to eventually carry himself in a more balanced frame.

The horse's conformation also may not lend itself to moving like a top dressage prospect, or a reining horse doing the perfect sliding stop, but the looser and more flexible you can keep him, the easier it will be for him to do things that may be a little bit of a stretch for him.

How to Address

Techniques to use:

Techniques	Page
Poll and Atlas Releases (Head Up, Head Down)	*pp. 45 and 51*
C7-T1 Release	*p. 92*
Hind Leg Releases	*p. 125*
Dorsal Arch	*p. 152*

As with stiff-backed or sore horses, the best way to work on ewe-necked or hollow-backed horses is first to release the poll and front end, then the hind end, the middle, or back. The whole body is involved in this issue. You may have to pay special attention to the poll and neck. As this condition has most likely developed for a while, it will take time to release tension that allows the horse to carry himself more naturally.

You will, however, probably see some improvement relatively quickly with these Techniques.

13. DOESN'T BEND IN THE BODY

Possible Primary Issues

This is another whole-body issue that can have developed from a number of primary issues. By going over the whole body you will have released the *Poll and Atlas, the C7-T1 Junction,* the *Sacroiliac Junction,* and released tension in the back and trunk. During the course of this bodywork, you should have been able to determine by his releases where restrictions were in his body that created an inability to bend. As the horse is often stiffer or more restricted when bending on one side than the other, it's important while determining what the primary issue, to compare side to side where the horse might have felt more restricted, sore, or shown more releases.

Here are some possibilities:

- *Restricted shoulders:* The horse's thoracic vertebrae do not naturally provide a lot of bend. Releasing tension in the shoulders and withers will often help a horse's ability to bend more in the front end.

- *Restricted range of motion in lumbar section:* The lumbar section is the most flexible area of the horse's back. Restriction there can inhibit "bend."

- *Saddle fit:* It's also important to make sure that the saddle fits the horse as well or better than it fits the rider. Improper saddle fit can affect movement of the shoulder, withers, lumbar area, and back.

- *Poll and atlas:* Tension or restriction in the poll and atlas affects everything.

How to Address
Techniques to use:

Techniques	Page
All Front and Hind End Techniques	*pp. 33–142*
All Back Techniques	*pp 143–158*

14. BUCKING, RUSHING, AND OTHER BEHAVIORAL AND TRAINING ISSUES

Possible Primary Issues

Often bucking and rushing are pain-related rather than training issues, especially when they show up in performance horses or horses that have already been trained through these behaviors.

The list of possible primary issues is long. Here are a few examples:

- A sore back due to any number of reasons, such as poor saddle fit that causes acute severe discomfort or accumulative chronic discomfort.

- Physical problems such as kissing spines or arthritis.

- Soreness in other parts of the body.

- Pain due to issues in the feet or legs.

- Pain or anticipation of pain, in general.

Bucking is often associated with a sore back, but can also be a reaction to pain or soreness elsewhere. This is one reason that going over the whole body is a good idea when dealing with this behavior.

You can begin the process of determining where the pain might be by correlating *what* you are asking the horse to do, with *when* he begins to buck or rush. For example, if the horse bucks after landing a jump, something that hurts upon land-ing might be the issue. This might include sore front feet, withers, or back.

Rushing can occur *while* the horse is feeling pain or discomfort, but can also happen *in antici-pation* of pain. For example, rushing in anticipa-tion of canter can occur when the horse's stifle has a tendency to lock during this gait, or if it is sore and bothers him at the canter.

It will also help determine what the issue is by making a note of *where* soreness or restriction occurs in the body during the course of the body-work. By collecting the data of *what, when, and where,* and putting pieces of the puzzle together, you may get a clue as to what is causing the behavior.

When you have a serious enough bucking or rushing problem on your hands, it is probably a good idea to consult a vet to rule out the possibil-ity of a serious physical issue before trying to train through the behavior.

How to Address

See Tables of Techniques in Problems 1, 3, 5, 8, 10 and 12.

Bucking: Begin by focusing on the scapula, with-ers, and back, taking note of anything that may have something to do with the bucking. During the course of going through the bodywork, if you determine there could be a primary cause for whatever you find, you have something that can be addressed.

Rushing: The problem could be in front, behind, or in between. When riding, if you can determine what precipitates the rushing, it may give you a

---

Case Study

I have a driving mare that used to rush before we approached the base of a hill. I knew that she would get sore behind when we drove because I didn't work her regularly enough and she was under-con-ditioned. She would anticipate the soreness associated with pulling up the hill and rush before the incline even began. Rather than turn it into a fight, I would give her some slack and as she became more fit, she rushed less. (I'm hoping this trend doesn't continue or *I* may end up pulling *her* up the hill!)

clue as to what end to focus on. Same as with bucking, pay attention to what shows up during the bodywork.

14. "HITCH" IN THE GAIT BEHIND; HIND LEG DRAGS A TOE

Possible Primary Issues
A chronic "hitch" can be the result of accumulated muscle tension in the hind end that causes structural imbalance or "misalignment." It creates more restricted movement on one side, or effectively makes one leg functionally shorter than the other, giving the horse a "hitch" in the movement. Often releasing tension in the sacroiliac junction, and lumbar area will get an improvement in the gait. How much improvement often depends on how entrenched the condition is.

Sometimes a hitch is caused by past trauma or injury. The injury, and the muscles that have had to compensate, have become contracted and tight. Regular bodywork can sometimes help balance things back up to some extent, although how much depends on how severe the injury was, and how long the imbalanced condition that resulted. Groin injuries take a long time to heal and if the horse is put back into work too soon, the affected muscles become pretty contracted. If a hitch has just started to develop, it would be a good idea to rule out a veterinary issue by consulting a vet. After the acute stage of an injury, releasing tension in the muscles will help them heal and retain their flexibility. If a new hitch is caused by developing unilateral tension then releasing the tension may stop it in its tracks.

How to Address
Techniques to use:

Techniques	Page
All Front and Hind End Techniques	*pp. 133–142*
All Back Techniques	*pp. 143–158*

It *always* helps to release the poll and atlas before working on the hind end. Apart from releasing tension in the area in general, in some cases, tension has accumulated in the atlas to such a degree that it creates a spasm in the gluteal muscles that may be part of the problem.

Lateral Rocking and *Dorsal Arch* will help release imbalances or restrictions in the lumbar and sacrolumbar area that may be part of the problem.

I have also had a lot of success with the *Hind End Release Points* when dealing with longstanding hind-end issues. It seems that older, more entrenched issues respond better to more subtle input. The horse's body has done such a good job of guarding and protecting an area for so long, that signals to the nervous system to move or let go *(Release Points)* work better than physically moving an area to get a release.

15. LESS AGILE AND FLEXIBLE, MORE LAZY AND UNWILLING

Possible Primary Issues
Stiff, sore, and restricted areas lead to a horse becoming more unwilling to move, which is often interpreted as laziness.

How to Address
Techniques to use:

Techniques	Page
All—The Full Monty!	*pp. 24–158*

You can improve both flexibility and comfort in older, arthritic horses just by asking for tiny increases in range of motion, and not forcing anything. You're just looking for an *improvement*. This is especially important with stiff and older horses so remember to *stop and soften* when you run into resistance. This will work wonders.

I don't know how many owners have told me after a gentle going over, how the next day their old horse is prancing around the pasture like a youngster.

Go slow, be patient with his limitations, and give him the full treatment from head to toe. Goodness knows, he deserves it!

CHAPTER 10

Bodywork
for Competition, Individual Breeds and Different Disciplines

Different equine sports and activities, in combination with different breed characteristics, result in a range of different considerations when doing this work. Below are some guidelines—what to look for overall, which areas tend to accumulate tension, and pre-event "loosening-ups." You will find issues particular to specific breeds due to factors such as conformation and disposition, and to different disciplines due to the nature of the sport.

As far as performance and body issues, these observations are just rules of thumb. The range of issues can apply to any horse in any sport.

Pre-Competition

When working on a horse before a competition or event, keep in mind you just want to loosen him up in general. We all have a tendency to want to "get 'er done" when we come across a problem, and "fix" it; however, just before the horse competes is not the time to do this.

Often, when a muscle has been extremely tight or restricted over a long period of time, it can be sensitive or sore when the tension lets go. This is best avoided right before competing. If you come across excessive resistance, pain, or restriction before an event, pass over it lightly. You can come back to it later. Keep in mind that the releases you get with Techniques can be deeper than you think. Every horse is different and some take a little longer to "recombobulate" than others, so allow yourself enough time before an event for this possibility.

There is a concern in some disciplines with getting the horse too loose. Dressage and reining horses—for example—need to keep a certain amount of functional muscle tightness in order to perform specific movements and hold the body in specific positions.

Individual horses will also respond differently to bodywork in general. Most will be more flexible and have more energy, but with some horses the looseness might come with a little laziness, and the horse might need to be pushed ahead more than usual.

When you work on a horse before an event, it is good to be familiar with him, his issues, and his response to the bodywork, for all of the above reasons. And if you're helping someone else with her horse before an event, keep in mind that if the horse doesn't do well you may be "asked" to take some responsibility for the poor showing. Just something to keep in mind.

STANDARD PRE-EVENT WORK

These are guidelines. Remember that the horse's responses play an important role in the work.

1. Go lightly over the poll, neck and lower neck with *Lateral Flexion* (p. 33). It's better to focus on the poll and atlas with this Technique rather than *Head Up* and *Head Down*—unless you know how the horse performs after these Techniques.

Case History

A Masterson Method Certified Practitioner and Instructor tells the story of a children's hunter that she did a little too much work on immediately before a class. It was the first time she had worked on the horse, and he had a lot to release as he demonstrated by yawning repeatedly throughout the bodywork.

The horse moved well through the class, and might have done a little better in points had it not continued yawning over the jumps!

---

2. *Scapula Releases:* If the horse can relax in the positions, let him (p. 62).

3. *Hind End Release Points:* No more than two or three minutes per side, unless the horse swats your hand away sooner (p. 111).

4. *Hind End Leg Releases:* Let the hind legs relax into the positions, if possible (p. 125).

5. *Lateral Rocking:* Take your time getting the horse to relax into the rocking (p. 143).

Note: *Unless the horse is familiar with the Dorsal Arch and it's part of his normal regimen, it's better to skip this one.*

TIPS

- Perform the Techniques gently, keeping in mind that you're only looking for an improvement, not to "fix" anything.

- If you run into excessive soreness or a restriction, pass over it lightly.

- Don't spend more than an hour working on a horse just before event time.

- Spend less time asking for *movements,* and more waiting for the horse to *relax into the positions.*

- You can spend longer on light work like the *Bladder Meridian Technique* and *Release Points* (pp. 24 and 111).

- Don't rush. The horse can tell when you're hurrying.

Different Breeds and Disciplines

HUNTERS AND JUMPERS

Pre-Event

Standard pre-competition work.

In General

Nowadays most horses in this discipline are the larger Warmbloods. They carry most of their weight on the *front end*. They land on the front end, so feet and legs are constant issues. Consequently, they accumulate a lot of tension in the poll and atlas, and in the lower neck and shoulder. In addition, most hunter-jumpers spend a lot of time in the stall—part of the job— but not necessarily the healthiest thing for the feet or for the horse's blood circulation. Weight has a big effect on the feet and due to the nature of this sport, hunters carry even more weight on the forehand. Sore feet equates with a sore neck and poll.

In the *hind end,* hocks and stifles are regular issues in hunter-jumpers. Generally, I find the tension in the hind end easier to release than in other sports such as dressage, but you will come across plenty of horses with hind-end issues. It's important to keep the lumbar area loose.

You will need to keep the mid-back loose, although you may not find as many back problems as you would think compared to some of the other riding disciplines. This may be because the rider spends a lot of time out of the seat, and the horse can carry himself in a more natural frame.

ENDURANCE HORSES

Pre-Event

Standard pre-event work. In addition, a little *Head Up* and *Head Down* can be worked in if you find the horse to be tense here (pp. 45 and 51) because during the ride, endurance horses have a little time to adjust to the bodywork if they need to. Spend time on *Release Point* work (p. 111). Make sure the hind end and back are loose.

In General

Endurance horses spend a lot of time in training so work pretty hard. Arabians (popular in this sport) can also be very alert and "mental" (in a good sense), so can hold a lot of tension in the poll and atlas. Their lighter weight makes it easier on the feet and legs, but they use them a lot so they can be sore just about everywhere. Hamstrings putting tension on the sacrum is pretty common, and the muscles of the back and lumbar area work hard and steadily.

Fortunately, in general, Arabian horses are easy to work on because of their size. You just have to have a little patience with their responses as they can be a little guarded by nature. (This is just a generalization. I know a lot of Arabian owners consider the breed "cuddly," but the "one-owner horse" can have a different view of a stranger like me coming into his stall the first time it happens.)

Endurance is one sport where being available to keep the horse loose at the holds *during* the event is helpful. I find it a good idea to leave the neck alone, but gentle *Front* and *Hind Leg Releases* are helpful, not only to keep the horse limber, but to feel when an area might be tensing up. Allowing the horse to rest for a minute in the *Farrier Position* alone can relieve a lot of tension in the sacrum, lumbar area and deeper muscles in the groin and psoas muscles.

Another thing that helps to keep tension from building in the back and hind end during the ride is to do the *Bladder Meridian*—using *air-gap* and *egg-yolk* pressures—especially on the back and lumbar area. Use the *Under-the-Tail Points* to release tension on the sacrum.

Anywhere the horse gives you a "blink" when working on the hind end is worth spending time on. Watch his eyes.

DRESSAGE HORSES

Pre-Event
Unless you are familiar with a particular horse and how he performs after bodywork, it is better that standard pre-event work be done at least three or four days before the event, especially when it is an important one.

In General
Dressage is very athletic and even the most well-balanced dressage horse can benefit from regular bodywork as he conditions for higher levels and new areas begin to "show up" as needing special attention. Bodywork is important if you want to keep the horse balanced, soft and moving forward.

Poll and Atlas
Particular attention should be paid to maintaining looseness and flexibility between the *occiput*

and *atlas* in the poll. If work isn't balanced, excessive tension can build there, affecting movement in the rest of the body.

Shoulder and Withers
As the neck, shoulders, and withers begin to strengthen, *Scapula* and *C7–T1 Releases* are important for progress to be made in this area.

Hind End
When the horse begins to get stronger in his hind end, movement in the pelvis and lumbar region needs to be maintained, and as the loin strengthens, lateral movement, too. *Lateral Rocking*, which progresses all the way from the pelvis up through the ribs into the back of the withers is particularly helpful with this, as is the *Dorsal Arch*. Loosening the sacrum using *Under-the-Tail* and other *Release Points* helps the horse release the increased tension from the developing gluteals and hamstrings. It's important to keep the pelvic structure and all its connections loose to help the horse "come through" from behind.

Training and Conditioning
Often training is pushed ahead at a faster pace than the level of conditioning can handle. When this happens, excessive tension develops in the hamstrings, sacrum, and eventually the muscles of the lumbar region. The dressage horse can become extremely tight in the poll, throatlatch and neck if the horse is over-ridden in front, leaving the hind end to fend for itself. When balanced self-carriage isn't allowed to develop naturally and evenly through the body, the front and hind ends have to work independently of each

other, and the back ceases being a part of the show. Focusing on the three key junctions—*Poll-Atlas Junction, Neck-Shoulder-Withers Junction,* and the *Sacroiliac Junction* will help keep the horse balanced. The *Head Up Technique* can be especially effective in the front end, and *Release Point* and *Hind Leg Release Techniques* that release tension on the sacroiliac are good behind.

EVENTERS

Pre-Event

Standard pre-competition work.

In General

By definition the goal of eventing is to develop a well-rounded equine athlete. You would expect to find the same range of issues in jumpers, dressage horses, and racing Thoroughbreds.

Overall, the eventers I've worked on seem all too often to share the same issues as those described in hunter-jumpers. I have also found that as they move up through higher levels of training they will develop similar issues in the hind end as dressage horses.

Many of the issues found in racing Thoroughbreds aren't necessarily found in eventers, possibly due to the later age at which event horses are trained and competed, and also possibly because of the more well-rounded conditioning afforded by cross-training in three different disciplines that make up eventing.

BARREL RACERS

Pre-Event

Standard pre-event work, with special attention given to the *poll, TMJ,* and *lower back.*

In General

Barrel horses sprint, stop, and turn in seemingly the same movement. The *Neck-Shoulder-Withers Junction* can be a consistent issue, along with ribs and back, especially just behind the withers. Tension or spasms in the *T18–L1 Junction* are common, possibly due to the "twisting" motion between hind and front ends required for the turns, and the power generated by the hind end that has to pass through this point. Transition points in the spinal column are common stress areas.

It's good to keep the poll and atlas loose, as they are so connected to flexibility in the rest of the body. Equally important with the barrel horse is the TMJ: When you find tension in the poll, it is likely you will find soreness in the TMJ and/or soreness in the feet.

THOROUGHBREDS—FLAT RACING

Thoroughbred racing is a demanding, professional sport. Thoroughbreds are put through serious conditioning. They start young, develop issues quickly, and have often received only minimal ground training when you get to them.

For racing Thoroughbreds, I've solicited contributions from Masterson Method Certified Practitioners who work in the Thoroughbred racing bodywork and health-rehabilitation fields. I'm hoping their perspectives will give you a good idea of what to expect.

Cyndi Hill is an Equine Sports Massage Therapist and Masterson Method Certified Practitioner who works on Thoroughbreds on the track.

Pre-Event

"Pre-event work I do is based to a large degree on the interaction with a particular horse, on a particular day. Working with Thoroughbreds is as much about establishing trust—reassuring the horse that I am not going to cause pain and learning his unique body-language vocabulary—as it is about identifying trouble spots. I find that I can get a more complete picture of what the horse needs by following his range of responses and 'staying under the radar,' thus avoiding any defensiveness caused by his anticipating pain."

In General

"I almost always find restriction deep in the shoulders and it usually extends into the base of the neck (*cervical trapezius* and *rhomboids*), down the pectorals, through the chest, (which can be very sensitive), and into the biceps. It doesn't matter where the "primary problem" is, it always ends up affecting the shoulders because they compensate for loss of impulsion by working harder and harder with the front end.

"I also find that many racehorses, due to the daily, ongoing physical demand of training and racing, tend to 'block out' body awareness and keep going however they can. Consequently, it is easy for them to become overwhelmed when they start to release and actually *feel* their body. Even if you are staying under the radar to get the release,

the release itself brings the focus to their body.

"Some develop hypersensitivity, some 'process' for a really long time, then don't want to be touched at all, and some go from calm and cooperative to defensive/aggressive. It is so important to really listen to the horse and recognize if he is becoming overwhelmed, end on a positive note, and work with him in several short sessions rather than a longer one.

"Beyond this, racehorse issues run the gamut, although the issues seem to be intensified due to their constant work."

Safety Note: I find that safety is really common, horse-handling sense. Contrary to popular belief, I find that most Thoroughbred racehorses are not hyperactive or aggressive. Many are young, and some are inexperienced with the concept of "personal space." Some have developed less-than-helpful coping mechanisms in response to pain or the anticipation of pain. The most important thing is to pay attention. Racehorses may be content, excited, tired, stressed, frustrated, annoyed, bored, anticipating pain, or working very hard not to feel pain. Their demeanor and expression can speak volumes. Listen to what the horse is telling you and believe him.

And below is what Geoffrey Pfeifer, Ph.D., N.P., a professional in the equine health field and a Masterson Method Certified Practitioner who works with racing Thoroughbreds on and off the track, has to add:

Pre-Event

"It takes a Thoroughbred quite a few days to adapt to having been worked on. Loosen up some tight muscles, get them to release physical and emotional tension, and the whole way they 'go' changes: their stride and their breathing. But if you do too much and they haven't had time for 'tightening' work or to get used to a new way of going, they're 'up the track' (they race terribly).

"The best way to pre-race a horse is to make sure he is not hurting when going into the race. In order to do this you need to do bodywork on him after each major work that he does for at least four to six weeks before the race. It will sometimes take two or three sessions to work the soreness out after the race so that he doesn't compound soreness on soreness and start getting sour. I've seen racehorses get so sour they stop in the middle of a race and pull up for no good reason. By being proactive you keep the soreness from stacking up and progressing from one area to others."

In General

"When looking at restrictions in Thoroughbreds, you're basically looking at the intersection of conformation with a number of factors: a progressive conditioning program (what the trainer asks the horse to do); training surface (synthetic, dirt, turf); jockey; nutrition; and physical-recovery program (if any).

"When the exercise jockey has poor balance, he'll exacerbate problems in the horse's shoulders and withers.

"In the United States, the typical Thoroughbred in training will never turn to the right while running, or even when being hot-walked. This produces common tension patterns that ultimately produce what has been called 'race-track lameness': a tension pattern from the left upper neck to the lower neck that continues down the left leg. Typically, the left side of the neck is worse than the right in the Thoroughbred on the track, resulting in the right hind end being worse than the left. Low back soreness is very common depending on how tightly coupled the horse's conformation is.

"The typical *dirt-track* 'profile' is tension starting in the upper neck and progressing down. As the horse keeps running with this tension pattern, the soreness progresses to the shoulders and withers, and then to the hind end and low back. Tension builds in the neck, the horse's stride shortens and control of the feet decreases, and he's poised to break down. The *synthetic-track* profile includes more low-back and hind-end problems early in the training process as compared to the dirt track."

Safety Note: As far as safety goes I am always adjusting my position based on "Where should I be if...." Never think that you are safe or that a horse can't kick you "from there." When you're dealing with green, poorly schooled two-year-old Thoroughbred racehorses, you've got to be mindful and careful. When they get worried they may try to pin you against the stall wall (the horse's second survival response is to "push against" or brace). Getting them to step backward is the most submissive movement for them, so if you're having trouble getting cooperation, stop and get them to step backward. Then move them forward, then backward again.

If you do this every five to ten minutes while working on them, it will change your entire relationship with them. They will start licking and "smacking" and start working with you to release tension rather than trying to assert their dominance. Letting them continue to exert their dominance can be dangerous while you are in the stall. Pay attention to the signs and if you feel the need to stop and do some ground-manners work, do so.

"When you handle them properly, the trainer will often notice that the horse's demeanor has changed and he is easier to work with. Most racing barns don't have enough grooms, skilled riders and assistant trainers to adequately school and train a racehorse, so it might pay to get your hands dirty and do yourself a favor by schooling him.

"Stay safe in the stall and good racing luck!"

STANDARDBREDS— HARNESS RACING

Pre-Event

Standard pre-event work can be done closer to the competition with Standardbreds than with, for example, Thoroughbreds. Standardbreds are bred and trained for stamina as well as speed, and warmup work done with the horse before the race is substantial.

In General

Standardbreds are some of the hardest-working horses in competitive equine sports. They condition hard for speed and stamina and their careers can be much longer than racing Thoroughbreds. Regular bodywork can lessen the effects of concussion on the feet and legs. The stress of high-speed trotting and pacing on the feet and legs can be high. Consequently, tension in the poll,

atlas and neck can become severe, often to one side more than the other, due to the natural tendency of the horse to favor one side more as well as the nature of track racing.

Fortunately harness racers can be conditioned in both directions on the track. When unilateral tension in the poll and neck develops, steering the sulky during the race can become an issue, which can get dicey during "rush hour." Pay special attention to these areas, but don't get carried away with the poll too close to the race. As with Thoroughbred racing, a regular regimen of bodywork is a very good pre-event strategy.

If you can also keep the sacrum, hamstrings, sacrolumbar junction and muscles of the lumbar loose, it will help with tension that develops along the topline from the poll to the tail as a result of the horse going in over-checks with the head high, which can also create tension in the back.

Auxiliary equipment such as head poles are designed to keep a trotter or pacer in a certain desired position (keep his neck/head from bearing to the right/left). If head poles are being used there is probably a steering issue and you will find considerable stiffness of the neck to both or one direction, tension in the TMJ, and especially in the poll area. Releasing tension and restriction in the poll and neck can lessen the need to use head poles.

I must differentiate between trotters and pacers. Pacers are unique in that they are one of three four-legged mammals (the other two are the camel and giraffe) that move both legs on the same side at the same time. Pacers carry slightly more weight on their front end than other horses. Their success in racing particularly depends on the flexibility of their shoulders. One-sided issues don't seem to be as prevalent as you might think, although there are enough issues with harness racers, in general, to keep you busy.

AMERICAN SADDLEBREDS

Pre-Event

As with dressage horses, unless you are familiar with the particular horse and how he performs after bodywork, it is better that the standard pre-event work is done at least three or four days beforehand, especially when it is an important competition. (As mentioned, regular bodywork is the best pre-event strategy.)

In General

The repetitive motion of horses that are trained to show with animated gaits can create noticeable muscle-tension patterns in different areas. These horses use muscles a lot more in some areas, and a lot less in others. These sports are very athletic and hard on feet and legs. Shoeing changes to enhance gaits can put a lot of stress on the feet and legs, as well, so you may find higher amounts of tension in the poll, upper neck, and TMJ. Action of the gaits in front works the muscles of the neck and shoulders, and hock and stifle action behind creates tension in the hamstrings and on the sacrum. This tension, when released, makes the requirements easier and more comfortable for the horse.

Body carriage affects neck and shoulders as well as the topline all the way through the muscles of the mid-back, lumbar, sacrolumbar, sacrum and hamstrings. Tail-sets used to accentuate tail carriage can create even more tension in the topline.

Overall, things to look for are higher amounts of tension in the poll/TMJ/upper neck; lower neck; limitations of both lateral flexion and rotation in the lumbar region; and high tension in the sacrum and hamstrings.

Other than all that you won't find a lot going on!

QUARTER HORSES—REINING, CUTTING, OTHER WESTERN SPORTS

Pre-Event

Unless you are familiar with how the horse performs after loosening the hind end, *do not* do *hind-end* work prior to an event because the horses need some tension in their hind end to "hold" the deep stops (see p. 188).

In General

Quarter Horses can be very well-muscled and compact, and sometimes a little stoic as far as bodywork is concerned. Their structure is comprised of a lot of short bones embedded in solid muscle. It helps to be patient when waiting for responses and not to expect large, fluid ranges of motion and movement as you go through the Techniques. This doesn't mean you are not getting releases of tension. What you don't see while working on the horse, you will see in improved performance.

In addition, as a result of some modern breeding preferences, some Quarter Horses' feet can be proportionally a little small for their stouter bodies. Tender feet equates tension in the poll and neck, so don't let their stoicism fool you when you get to the poll, neck, and shoulders. Of course, there's a lot to the Quarter Horse's hind end, too, but I find that they respond to the all of the *Hind End Techniques* very well.

The following insights on reining, cutting, and reined cow horses are contributed by Tamara Yates. Tamara is a Masterson Method Certified Practitioner and Instructor, and shows horses in these disciplines.

REINING HORSES

"Reining horses need to have their lumbar, SI, and pelvis and hip joints kept flexible as they build strength in the hindquarters for the sliding stops. The *Hind Leg Releases* are vital, in particular, the position of the leg to the back resting on the toe and asking the horse to sink into the hip, thereby releasing the psoas. Regular releases of the entire *hind end* are invaluable for maintaining soundness.

"More important, and perhaps less obvious, is the need to keep a reining horse's shoulders and withers loose. Reiners often travel with their head and neck low, but their shoulders must be 'up' in order to perform the maneuvers required of them. Loose shoulders are a major part of a well executed sliding stop as well as a fluid and fast turnaround. Releasing tension in the Scapulae and C7–T1 is exceptionally helpful for increasing performance."

CUTTING HORSES AND REINED COW HORSES

"Cutting horses' and reined cow horses' stifles and hocks are used more than in any other discipline. The torque experienced on hocks is significant and the lateral movement of the stifle is almost constant in the cutting pen. Between events, getting these horses loose throughout the pelvis, in particular the sacrum and the hip joint (along with the gluteals) is a priority.

Emphasizing the hip drop with the *Hind Leg Release Down and Back,* wiggling the hock and stifle back and forth with the toe resting on the ground helps to maintain hock and stifle soundness. Maintaining lateral flexibility in the lumbar vertebra also relieves stress on the stifles and hocks. These horses also need loose shoulders and C7–T1 freedom to make the sweeping moves necessary to hold a cow. Keeping fluidity in the neck with *Lateral Cervical Flexion* moves earns points for cutting horses for 'eye appeal.' Like reiners, however, you need to be careful how close to an actual event a full-body workout is performed. Recognize that some tension is needed in the hind end to hold the ground while working the cattle.

***

Note: *Reining horses and reined cow horses—on the day of a show, or even the day before, DO NOT do a complete release of the groin and gluteals as the horses need some tension in the hind end to "hold" the deep stops. These releases are important between shows and during conditioning and training. Every horse is different, but often if the adductors and abductors are too relaxed as the horse goes into the show pen, the stops are harder for him to hold.*

THE DIFFICULT, HIGH-STRUNG, OR REACTIVE HORSE

The key to handling is in:
- The softness of your hand.

- The firmness of your hand.

- Timing.

Softness

When you place your hand on the horse and he feels that you're going to grab him, he's going to pull away. If your hand is soft (and you don't react to his initial reaction by grabbing), he will relax a bit. In fact, he will probably be surprised that you didn't react to his initial reaction by grabbing.

If you can keep your hand soft, nine out of ten, the horse will trust you enough to stay as relaxed as he possibly can. This goes back to the principle that if you give him nothing to brace against, he will stop bracing. When you feel the horse even slightly start to brace, soften your hands and yield a tiny bit.

So, you ask, if I yield every time he braces or moves, how am I going to get anything done?

Firmness

This is where the firmness comes in. You have to let him know with your handling that he has the option of yielding to the space you give him. You create a boundary with your hand that he can stay relaxed within (keep him "in the neighborhood"). This boundary is the tiny bit that you gave him when you softened and yielded at his initial bracing.

So, you now ask, how do I let him know that he has the option of yielding to this boundary?

Timing

Timing makes this all work. You can be firm with the horse if you are prepared to yield to him immediately when he does what you ask. One thing I've noticed about being firm is that whenever I grab, hold, force, or brace with my hand, it is almost never for more than half a second. I mean literally *half a second*… half of "one alligator."

If you use this one trick of never bracing for more than half a second, you'll find that most of your resistance problems will be solved. To get a good feel for this, practice the "Try this at home!" exercise on p. 76.

It is important, though, that you not take your hand off the horse when you yield, or every time he throws his head. Otherwise, he will quickly (in about two seconds) learn to throw his head to remove your hand. This goes for any time the horse shows his discomfort at what you are doing.

Frequently Asked General Questions

■ *How long before I can ride my horse after bodywork?*

■ *What the best thing to do for the horse after a bodywork session?*

After a session, the best thing for the horse is to be able to move around comfortably. Hand-walking, a relaxed ride on a loose rein, or turnout are good choices. If you have the option, turnout is ideal. The idea is to let the horse's body move and feel what's been released. But if your horse is on an exercise or training schedule and must be ridden that day, it is a good idea to give him as easy a ride as possible. If you start asking for work too soon, the tension will return before the horse's body has a chance to integrate or process the release.

Usually one day is enough, but if you get on and the horse is uncomfortable, it usually means he needs a little more time. This may be the case if he had a lot of tension in the body and you worked on him for a long time.

For the best results, resist the temptation to hop on and "see how he goes" right after the bodywork.

■ *Should I work on the horse before riding, or after?*

In my experience, with this method of bodywork, it is easier for the horse to release tension when the muscles are *not* in an active state. This means it is better to work on the horse when he is "cold," or *before* he works out. This differs from stretching muscles in this respect, which should be warm when done.

■ *When is the best time of the day to work on the horse?*

Anytime there is a little peace and quiet around the barn, but you'll be surprised how relaxed and calm the horse might become with a lot going on, especially if you don't react to the noise around you. I find the evenings after feeding time when everybody's done for the day to be good, but I'm a night person.

■ *How long should I work on my horse?*

If you are taking your time and not doing too much in one go, then two hours is not too long to work on your horse. If you are doing a lot, you should make the session a little shorter. There is a lot going on with the horse's nervous system with these releases, so when you are getting huge releases, be aware that the horse might need a rest. Sometimes the horse will just tell you that he has had enough. You need to differentiate between this and horses that are uncomfortable with the whole idea of releasing, or that just need a moment to process. You will know you've gone too long when the horse simply stops giving you responses.

■ *How often should I work on my horse? How much is too much?*

This depends on things such as how much you do on the horse in one session, or how much tension the horse accumulates between sessions. For general guidelines, when the horse is competing or training hard, two times a week is okay. When the horse is not worked hard, yet has issues from the past that you want to help him clear up, you might work on him a couple of times the first week, then once a week until you feel that he's doing better, then once a month.

It won't take long for you to be able to tell what the horse's body is telling you. You'll be able to feel when the tension is gone, and when there is nothing more to release. When the horse stops giving you responses, either his nervous system needs a break, or there is nothing more there to release.

When you first work on your horse, you will often feel like there is more to do. It's good to give the horse at least two or three days between two sessions. After that, as I said above, it's better not to work on the horse more than two times a week. This is something you will get a feel for after doing some of this bodywork.

■ *Do I always have to perform the entire sequence?*

No. Go by what's comfortable for you and the horse, or by what areas of performance you are interested in improving.

■ *I am short and my horse is tall. How do I perform the Techniques effectively?*

The only Techniques that you think may be difficult are the ones that involve the head. The key here is to get the horse to lower his head to you. If he tries to keep out of reach, it's probably because he is trying to guard against you going there, which means he's uncomfortable there. So when this happens, move somewhere else.

With the head, you would start either with *Leg Releases,* or with gentle *Lateral Flexion* at the lower neck, and *very* softly work your way up. If he starts to tense up, yield and soften to make sure he's comfortable with it, but try *not* to take your hand off his nose. If you can't get anywhere near his head, move on to other Techniques and at some point he will start to relax into it.

It's important not to get into a hurry to accomplish any one thing or the horse will sense it and become worried.

It's not the best idea to stand on something unless your horse is comfortable enough with it to stand completely still. If he's that comfortable, you're better off asking him to bring his head down to you.

What if my horse is "mouthy" or keeps nipping at me or the handler?

If you are working on the horse alone and he is mouthy or nippy, tie him with enough room to bend and flex as much as he can, without reaching you. You can let the rope out the farther back you are working, and shorten it when you are closer to the front. Be sure to tie him safely. If you are in a stall, tie him to a piece of baling twine, or something that will break if he pulls back hard. You don't want him to break something in the stall and fall back, and you really don't want to be in the stall with a horse that won't give up trying to break away. And lastly, pulling back on something hard is often the cause of poll problems to begin with.

If he is bothering the person holding him, then have the handler run the lead rope through something and hold the end while standing away from the horse where he can't reach her.

What if he is a constant cribber or keeps chewing on the lead rope?

It is just plain difficult to read the responses of a cribber, but not necessarily impossible. Just keep on working and watching and see what happens. Sometimes it's when the horse stops chewing, cribbing, or fidgeting that a change is happening. Or the horse might all of a sudden break loose and start yawning, licking, chewing, snorting. If you just keep doing what you're doing you'll start to see through the fidgety behavior. Have more patience than the horse.

What if he won't hold still?

If he's already tied and he won't hold still or keeps stepping from side to side, continue doing whatever you were doing with your hand on him, and just step from side to side with him, or walk with him. Once he realizes that by taking a step your hand's not going anywhere, he'll usually stop walking. If not, you can be firm with him, as long as you relax when he yields to your request. Often, when you soften whatever you were doing, the horse stops fidgeting or moving. Don't get frustrated with a fidgety horse. Fidgeting means it's working, and if you stay with it, more often than not, you'll get a release.

When he's not tied and won't hold still, if it helps you get the work done, then tie him.

I learned a different type of massage or bodywork. Will the Masterson Method interfere with it, or vice versa? Should I stop doing it?

Not necessarily. This method of reading the horse's responses can be integrated into, or used in any modality.

Can I work on my pregnant mare?

This is something you should consult your vet. Generally, it is not good to do any type of massage on a pregnant mare before there is a fetal heartbeat (the first month) or during the last month, especially with the *Hind End Release Points* that we use.

■ **Do I still need a chiropractor if I use the Masterson Method?**

If you can't position *yourself* properly when handling the feet and legs, you may!

As far as *your horse* needing a chiropractor, you should be able to determine this yourself after using this Method for a while. Different horses respond differently to different "inputs." There are different types of chiropractic out there as well. Some horses respond better to gentler methods, and for some, a good old-fashioned adjustment is just what they need. If you feel that your horse responds well to chiropractic, you should continue. The Masterson Method can be integrated into just about any modality. Many horse people are interested in learning alternative methods of keeping their horses healthy. This one may suit you and your horse.

■ **I understand the Techniques and tried them on my horse, but still feel I need more instruction. Is there a way to learn this Method hands-on?**

You're probably doing better than you think, but if you feel you need hands-on instruction, contact us at www.mastersonmethod.com for more information on our training programs.

■ **Can I perform this type of work on other equines like miniatures, donkeys, or mules?**

Yes! These Techniques are safe and effective on any type of equine. (Running shoes are recommended when working on wild Mustangs and Zebras.)

■ **How soon after foaling can I work on my mare?**

Consult the veterinarian who is following the mare's pregnancy.

■ **My horse's nose starts running when I work on him. What does this mean?**

Get used to this happening. It's going to a lot, sometimes right away as tension in the poll and atlas releases and the sinuses start to relax. This is a good sign that tension is releasing. I just forgot to put it under the *Release Responses* to look for!

■ **My horse lay down and went to sleep for several hours after the bodywork. Is this something to worry about?**

Not unless you are trying to ride him. This is another thing that can happen with horses that have held a lot of tension in their body. It seems to occur more to young horses. At one seminar, the students did a lot of work on a two-year-old that had a lot of tension in the poll. The horse lay down in the stall and was out for almost two hours. I was starting to wonder myself, if everything was okay, that is until feeding time, when he got up.

At another seminar, a young horse lay down in the center of the paddock we were working in, completely oblivious to the human traffic around him. It was a lesson to me how much tension a young horse, not yet even ridden, can accumulate due to factors such as his conformation, or something that may have happened to him in the pasture one day, or during foaling.

■ *Is it okay to work with the horse right after he had his grain?*

I haven't noticed any ill-effects of doing bodywork on the horse after eating. If you notice that there is something not quite right, then stay on the safe side and wait.

■ *Can he eat while I'm working on him?*

No. Food is the one thing that will interfere with your reading his responses, and interfere with him releasing. If he does want to eat, take the food out of the stall, or tie him if he pretends he's starving and needs to clean up every little bit of hay.

■ *Is there a Technique I can use to help a colicking horse?*

The *Under-the-Tail Points,* or any of the *Hind End Release Points* that don't obviously bother the horse will help the horse to relax. Some colicky horses respond better than others. These Techniques work well when used at the first signs of colic, but will be less effective the more severe the condition becomes. By no means use this as a substitute for veterinary attention if you feel that the horse needs a vet.

■ *My husband/wife/friend/sister/trainer thinks this is a bunch of hocus-pocus. Is he/she right?*

He/she may be. But if it gets results, do it!

APPENDIX 2

Active Stretches

In addition to the bodywork exercises described in this book, *active stretches* are a beneficial addition that can be easily incorporated into your daily routine.

You can find a number of different descriptions of *carrot stretches* online or in books such as Hillary Clayton's *Activate Your Horse's Core* (Sporthorse Publications, 2008).

Here are some of our favorite stretching exercises:

- To the outside of the front hoof

- To the shoulder/elbow

- Bending around the human to the point of hip

- To the girth line

- To the knee

- Down and back

- Down and forward

Keep in mind that when you bring the horse's nose in close to the point of the shoulder or the chest, that he is flexing the poll, atlas, and upper neck. As you bring the head farther around to the flank, hip, or legs you are flexing the area of the lower neck.

You may also notice that the horse sometimes flattens his head or turns it sideways (corkscrews) when he brings his head around. As mentioned in *Lateral Cervical Flexion* (p. 33), this will happen when the vertebrae of the upper neck become stiff, and rather than flexing laterally—or side-to-side—the horse flattens his neck and flexes them dorsally—that is, up and down—but on a sideways plane. You can help him to flex a little more laterally by guiding his nose out and around more, and by lifting slightly on his nose or noseband as you do it.

APPENDIX 3

Contraindications

These Techniques are intended to enhance performance in the healthy horse. This bodywork is not meant to treat any type of disease or be used as a substitute for veterinary care and treatment. If you are in doubt about the physical health of your horse, please consult your vet, especially in case of:

ARTHRITIC HORSES

Light bodywork can make the arthritic horse more comfortable. If your horse is being treated by a veterinarian for arthritis, consult him/her regarding bodywork on the horse.

PREGNANT MARES

Do not perform bodywork on pregnant mares in the first month or the last trimester. Check with your treating veterinarian.

ACUTE INJURIES

Bodywork is not indicated on horses with injuries at the acute stage. Heat and swelling are signs of this.

INFECTIOUS DISEASES (LYME, EPM)

Gentle bodywork may be a good way to support the healing of a horse with Lyme disease or EPM during the course of treatment. Consult your veterinarian.

HIVES

Horses that suffer from allergies or hives can be especially sensitive to touch. Experiment with levels of touch and—if you find that your horse's condition worsens with bodywork—stop and consult your veterinarian.

HORSES ON STALL REST

Ask your veterinarian before performing bodywork on a horse on stall rest. Depending on his condition, gentle bodywork can be an excellent way to keep him supple, flexible, in good spirits with his blood circulation going. Be aware that the horse may not be able to support himself on three legs during *Leg Releases* if the reason he's on stall rest is a foot or leg issue.

Note: *The above list is by no means complete. Again, if in doubt regarding the health condition of your horse, consult your veterinarian.*

APPENDIX 4

Recommended Reading

The Equus Illustrated Handbook of Equine Anatomy, Volume I by Susan E. Hakola and Ronald J. Riegel (Primedia Equine Network, 2006)

Horse Structure and Movement by R.H. Smythe, MRCVS, and revised by Peter Gray, MVB, MRCVS (J.A. Allen, 1992)

The Horse's Muscles in Motion by Sara Wyche (Crowood Press, 2002)

The Horse's Pain-Free Back and Saddle-Fit Book by Joyce Harman DVM, MRCVS (Trafalgar Square Books, 2004)

Physical Therapy and Massage for the Horse by Jean-Marie Denoix and Jean-Pierre Pailloux (Trafalgar Square Books, 2001)

Release the Potential: A Practical Guide to Myofascial Release for Horse & Rider by Doris Kay Halstad and Carrie Cameron (Half Halt Press, 2000)

True Unity by Tom Dorrance and edited by Milly Hunt Porter (Give-It-A-Go Enterprises, 1987)

Tug of War: Classical versus Modern Dressage by Dr. Gerd Heuschmann (Trafalgar Square Books, 2007)

Understanding the Horse's Back by Sara Wyche (Crowood Press, 1998)

The Western Horse's Pain-Free Back and Saddle-Fit Book: Soundness and Comfort with Back Analysis and Correct Use of Saddles and Pads by Joyce Harman, DVM, MRCVS (Trafalgar Square Books, 2008)

Acknowledgments

For anyone thinking of taking on the challenge of accumulating whatever body of knowledge he or she might have and writing a book, let this be fair warning that it's nowhere near a one-man job—neither in the accumulation of the knowledge, nor the writing of the book.

I'd like to thank those involved, wittingly or unwittingly, in the accumulation of knowledge that this book presents:

As a young horse trainer, Val Lowe gave me the opportunity to get into horses on a working basis (in other words, "a job"). Two talented equine massage therapists from Texas introduced me to the basics of putting your hands on the horse at a show in Estes Park. It was while watching them that I started noticing subtle signs from the horse that indicated something good was happening.

A strong inspiration to me along the way was an old-time New Zealand horse chiropractor who'd practiced his trade for 40 years. He'd learned from another old chiropractor who'd practiced his trade for 40 years. My time spent following and watching him was a little shorter—about 10 days—but during that time I learned one or two key elements that made the difference and saw things that inspired me to keep on learning.

I'd also like to thank my friend and partner Bill Stanton, of Bill Stanton Integrated Equine Bodywork. Bill and I were both inspired by the same unnamed chiropractor. By including me in his successful practice, Bill has given me the opportunity to continue learning on thousands of horses over the years. Thanks, Bill.

In 2006 Valerie Kanavy asked me to accompany the US Endurance Team to the World Equestrian Games in Aachen, Germany. I thank her for giving me that opportunity and for her support since.

Without a doubt my biggest inspiration came, of course, from the horses—they taught me everything there is to know about the Masterson Method…up to this point. I'm sure they're holding some back to share later.

For helping me overcome the unexpected challenge of putting a book together, I thank:

Stefanie Reinhold, my co-author, for her organizational skills and thorough knowledge of the subject. Tamara Yates, Geoffrey Pfeifer, and Cyndi Hill, for their contributions regarding working on horses of different disciplines. And Joe Stanski and Geoff Northridge, for their willingness to provide critical photography at a moment's notice.

Marcus Brauer in Germany, for the bulk of the excellent photography. Also in Germany, my friends Daniela Wallraf-Pflug and Renate Frantzen, who kindly helped organize the photo shoot on location and kept us well-fed and in good spirits with their generous hospitality. Thank you to the friendly, welcoming owners of Gut Neuhaus in Aachen (www.gut-neuhaus.de), as well as the helpful horse owners there, who patiently volunteered their time and their handsome horses: Michael Scholz,

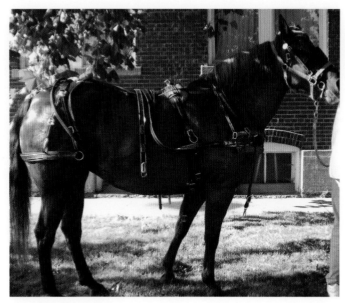

My trusty Annabelle.

Manuela Mirgartz, Therese Scheins, and Martina Fischer. And, in the United States I would like to thank Melissa Worthington for the use of her horse Chase.

To my local pub, and Annabelle, who faithfully got me there and back safely, whenever the need arose.

And finally to my partner and wife Conley, without whose moral support and inspiration I would be sitting on a tailgate by the side of the road holding a cardboard sign that reads, "Will work on horses for food."

Index

Page numbers in *italics* indicate illustrations.

Standardbred horses, 186–187

Stay phase, of cycle of interactions, 11–12, 30

Stepping back, 40, 42, 131

Stepping under, lack of, *163*, 168–169

Sternomandibular muscles, 93

Stiffness, vs. pain, 162. *See also* Bending problems

Stifle joints
    in performance/competitive disciplines, 162, 165, 181, 188
    release points of, *112*, 120–121, *120–121*

Stimulus, touch as, 5–6

Stretching, 9, 156, 192, 197

Stringhalt, 136

Stubbornness, vs. pain response, 14–15, 73, 74

Suppleness, of poll, 145

Supraspinaous ligament, 35, *35*, 45, 110, *110*

Survival instincts, 3–4

Suspension, 64–65

Symmetry. *See* Asymmetry

Synthetic track tension profile, 185

Tack
    bits, *163*, 167
    as cause of tension, 160
    in harness racing, 186
    saddles, 35, 160, 175

Tail anatomy, 144, *144. See also* Under-the-Tail release points

Tall horses, working with, 193

Teeth, grinding of, 59. *See also* Dental issues

Tension and tension patterns
    forelimb pain and, 35
    in hind end, 110–111, 133
    performance and, 4–5
    in race horses, 185
    range-of-motion release of, 15, 56, 147

softening of touch level and, 7

Thoracic vertebrae, 100, 143, *144*, *145*, 151

Thoroughbred race horses, 183–186

Timing
    of work/exercise after bodywork, 170, 192, 196
    of yielding of touch, 7, 189

Ting Points, 29, *29*

Toes
    dragging of, *163*, 177
    holding horse's foot by, 83, *83*, 88, *88*

Topline, contracted, 168–169

Touch
    correlation with behavior, 31
    vs. firmness in handling, 189
    levels of, 6–7, 124
    response and, 5–6, 10–12
    speed of hand movement in, 12, 28
    timing and, 189

Track surfaces, in racing, 185

Training issues, 175–177, 182–183, 185–186

Transition points, of spine, 151, 183

Transverse processes, 144, *145*

Treats, 17, 196

Trot, hard to sit, 172

Trotters, vs. pacers, 186

Tuber coxae, 106, *109*

Tuber sacrales, 105, *109*

Turnout, after bodywork, 170, 192

Tying tips, 17–18, *18*, 31, 194

Under the Scapula–C7-T1 Junction Release
    goals and effects, 92–93
    step-by-step, 93–96, *94–96*
    tips and what ifs, 96–99

Understanding the Horse's Back (Wyche), 145

Under-the-Tail release points, *112*, 114–117, *115–117*, 123, 182

Unilateral resistance, 169

Vertebrae. *See* Spinal column

Waiting
    in cycle of interactions, 11–12, 30
    for release, 40, 42, 131

Withers. *See also* Neck-Shoulder-Withers Junction
    anatomy of, 63, *63*, 92–93, *100*
    Check and Release Technique, 100–103
    in pre-event bodywork, 182

Work. *See also* Performance problems; Pre-competition bodywork
    as cause of tension, 161
    timing of, following bodywork, 170, 192, 196

Work areas, 16–17, 19

Working the Hind End from the Bottom
    goals and effects, 104–105, 109–111
    Hind Leg Down and Forward, 125–136

Working the Hind End from the Top
    goals and effects, 104–105, 109–112
    release points in, 112–124

Wyche, Sarah, 145

Yates, Tamara, 188

Yawning, 9–10, *9*, 72, 180

Yielding
    of handler to resistance, 41, 76, 131–132
    of horse to handler, 19
    of touch level, 7, 13, 189

Young horses, 184, 195

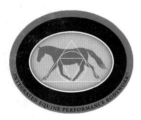

Further Resources & Contact Information

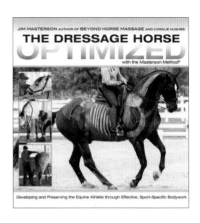

Additional instructions and visual aids for Masterson Method® Techniques can be found in the DVD and wall charts also entitled *Beyond Horse Massage*, the DVD set *Dressage Movements Revealed*, and the book *The Dressage Horse Optimized with the Masterson Method*, all available through www.mastersonmethod.com or Trafalgar Square Books (www.horseandriderbooks.com).

Masterson Equine Services also offers a progressive schedule of hands-on seminars and training certification courses in the Masterson Method. To learn more or to find a Masterson Method Certified Practitioner, go to www.mastersonmethod.com or call 641.472.1312.

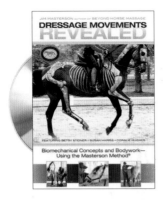

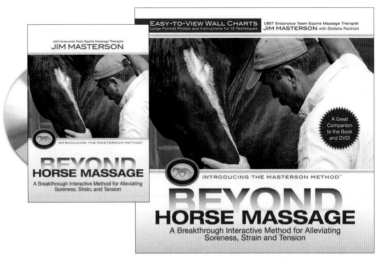